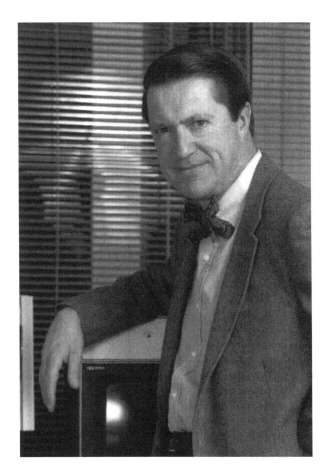

Dr. Thomas L. Petty
1932 – 2009

Thomas L. Petty, MD

Adventures

of an

Oxy-Phile$_2$

with Robert McCoy, BS, RRT, FAARC,
Louise Nett, RN, RRT, FAARC,
and Kay Bowen

Snowdrift Pulmonary Conference, Inc
Denver, Colorado

Manuscript Preparation and Review: Kay Bowen and Louise Nett
Book Design: Don Eastburn & Associates, Denver, Colorado
Mark Gelotte and Don Eastburn
www.doneastburn.com

Printed in the United States of America

ISBN978-0-615-37057-6

DEDICATION TO DR. THOMAS L. PETTY

We dedicate this book to Dr. Thomas L. Petty and all the patients he so loved. Dr. Tom dedicated his life to the medical profession so he could help others.

He was a hard working young boy with a paper route in Boulder, Colorado. That job led to work at the Boulder Camera newspaper. He learned a lot about writing for the public during that time. His mother, Eleanor, encouraged Tom to write. His Childhood Recollections book shows his gift for writing at an early age. Writing came easily to Dr. Tom. During his lifetime he wrote over 800 articles and 45 books. For information on his diverse medical interests see his curriculum vitae at www.drtompetty.org.

In addition to writing, he edited numerous projects. The one that was a challenge to Tom and his last secretary, Kay Bowen, was the annual *Yearbook of Pulmonary Disease* from 1992 to 1997. He and his good friend, Dr. Roger Bone, co-authored the first five books. When Roger became terminally ill, Tom took on this assignment by himself and was sole editor in 1997. The *Yearbook* reviews thousands of medical articles from the previous year to find significant ones to include. Tom was not only a prolific writer, but also an accomplished editor. Another major editing assignment was the *Seminars in Respiratory Medicine Journal*. He and his colleague, Dr. Reuben Cherniack at the National Jewish Health in Denver, were senior editors of that journal from 1979

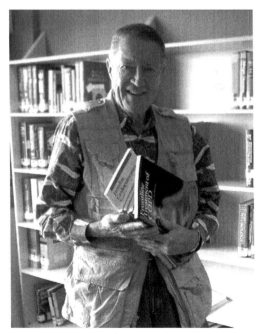

2002 Snowdrift

to 1986. Together Rueben and Tom made a great team in developing the training and research program for the University of Colorado and the National Jewish Health in Denver. Tom was also on the editorial board of 17 medical journals.

Tom enjoyed writing books, booklets, and pamphlets for patients. Tom and his friend and colleague, Louise Nett, co-authored their first book for patients in 1967, *For Those Who Live and Breathe.* The dedication in this book is relevant today. It reads:

> This book must be dedicated to our patients. These individuals living today have been a constant source of inspiration, new ideas, and hope for the others with emphysema and chronic bronchitis. These patients with tremendous courage have clamored for guidelines on how to live and breathe despite, often times, serious disease. They tell us more patients should be taught about what is known and understood concerning the care and rehabilitation of patients with emphysema and chronic bronchitis — thus we present this book to them.

In 1984 they again collaborated on a book for patients entitled *Enjoying Life With Emphysema.* In the seventeen years since the first book had been published, there had been a developing interest in pulmonary medicine. By this time, small pulmonary function machines were used in the outpatient clinics and the general hospital units. This advanced knowledge and the early diagnosis of pulmonary diseases led to earlier treatment. Pulmonary rehabilitation was catching on around the country. Long term oxygen therapy for patients with chronic lung disease was quite common in Colorado and other areas of the country where there were established pulmonary rehabilitation programs. The foreword of this book from 1984 could be used for this book today.

> The authors have captured the essence of the emphysema problem and expressed it in terms of the layman. They have conveyed important information about the nature of the emphysema problem, how patients are evaluated and treated, and how they can learn to cope with disease. It is hoped that some facets of this book will stimulate both physicians and patients to seek early identification of emphysema and early treat-

ment. An enlightened public can become a major force in reducing the social and economic impact of this important health problem.

Unfortunately, many of the dozens of short pamphlets for physicians and patients written by Dr. Petty in his early years are no longer available. These publications held a succinct message for physicians and patients alike. The titles tell of his interest in several major areas of pulmonary care: *Chronic Lung Disease – A Practical Office Approach to Early Diagnosis; Office Spirometry – For the Assessment of Pulmonary Disease – Practical Spirometry – For Office, Clinic, Workplace and Hospital; Maintenance Management for Chronic Pulmonary Disease – A Physicians' Guide; Save Your Breath – Advice for Patients and Family; Ambulatory Oxygen – Prescribing Home Oxygen for COPD.* This was also translated into Japanese and Italian.

Dr. Tom loved to write. He started his day very early and that is the time he said he could be most productive in this endeavor. He was blessed with very good secretaries who were as dedicated to his projects as he was. Some of the key secretaries were Jean Finleysen, Patty Way and Sandy Blegebron in the early years. From 1979 until 1989, Jeanne Cleary was his secretary. After Tom left the university, Jeanne continued to coordinate the Aspen Lung Conference, a project dear to Tom. This conference was named after him in 1990. While at Presbyterian/St. Luke's Medical Center, beginning in 1989, his secretary until his death was Kay Bowen. He often started his work day at five AM and Kay, his loyal secretary, was not far behind at six AM. If you Google his name be sure to say MD or you will get the singer Tom Petty. You will find a lot of information about him at various web sites including his own at www.drtompetty.org.

After the early morning phone calls to the East coast, he started writing. Then when the rest of the world was up and at it Tom made physician rounds. He was a real patient care doctor. He spent many hours in the hospital caring for sick critical care patients and making teaching rounds with young doctors. Afternoons were usually spent in the outpatient clinics or the private practice clinics. He would have been happy to see patients 12 hours or longer each day. Dr. Petty learned medicine in the old school. He based his diagnosis on the symptoms and history of the patient. The medical tests supplemented his knowledge and experience. He was like a detective in getting to the bottom of the patient's complaint. He often said a good doctor was like Columbo.

Dr Tom enjoyed visiting the pulmonary rehab program that Mary Burns directed in California at their yearly rally. He and Dr. Brian Tiep, along with Mary Burns, wrote three great pamphlets. One of these was "Essentials of Pulmonary Rehabilitation." These can be found on the web site http://www.perf2ndwind.org/Essentials. In addition the Letters From Tom written to the PEP Pioneers monthly over many years are archived on the web site. Kay Bowen and I hope to reproduce a hard copy book of some of these letters with current comments from friends and colleagues.

Starting in 2004, Dr Tom answered questions from patients on the American Association for Respiratory Care internet web site http://www.yourlunghealth.org under the column of "Ask Dr. Tom." He was always to the point with his responses. The American Association for Respiratory Care continues to keep this column active under the web site. Most of his archived answers can still be found there. He loved doing this as it kept him closely connected with patients. During this time he answered thousands of questions.

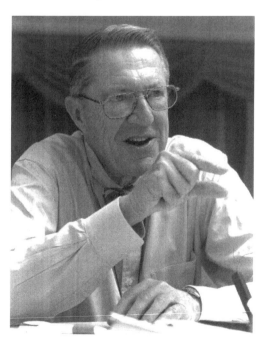

Dr. Petty teaching

Tom had many other interests in pulmonary medicine in addition to pulmonary rehab and LTOT oxygen. He was head of the training program for young pulmonary doctors. He and Dr. David Ashbaugh are credited with describing the acute respiratory distress syndrome (ARDS). Their sentinel paper on this topic led to exciting research over the last 43 years.

He was head of the Pulmonary Division at the University of Colorado from 1971 to 1983. His great joy was helping young pulmonary doctors find their particular niche in pulmonary medicine. Tom loved to teach and was proud of the fact that he taught in almost every state in the US and many foreign countries. Some credit him with starting modern day pulmonary medicine even though his original interest was in tuberculosis. In 2006 he was honored by the American College of Chest Physicians with the Legacy in Pulmonary Medicine Award. They considered him the Father of Pulmonary Medicine. After the tuberculosis unit at University of Colorado hospital closed, Tom focused his energies and interest in critical care and pulmonary rehabilitation.

During the last 14 years, he was a champion for early detection of COPD and the early detection of lung cancer. In 1996 he started a quarterly newsletter for pulmonary physicians, Lung Cancer Frontiers, in hopes that they would develop an interest in early diagnosis of lung cancer. The archives of the newsletter can be found on his website. In 2008 National Jewish Health in Denver took over the publication of the newsletter. Current issues can be found on their website http://www.nationaljewish.org/.

He founded a program for early detection for chronic obstructive lung disease called the National Lung Health Education Program (NLHEP) under the umbrella of the Snowdrift Pulmonary Conference, Inc. Tom felt that if physicians would only start doing simple pulmonary function tests in their offices, they would find patients with COPD early in the course of illness. Early diagnosis for most all diseases results in earlier treatment and that results in better care for patients. Today many medical equipment companies are producing simple pulmonary function machines for the primary care doctor's office. He was pleased to play a small part in initiating a change in physician practice. The NLHEP is now a program of the American Association for Respiratory Care for more information on early detection. Check resources at http://www.nlhep.org. Dr. Petty believed that all patients with respiratory symptoms should have a lung test.

Dr. Roger Mitchell, the Chief of Pulmonary Medicine, was Tom's mentor in 1965. Roger had organized seven Aspen Lung Conferences. There was none scheduled for 1965. Tom thought there should be at least one on the treatment aspects of COPD. Roger did not object but said there was no money for such a meeting. Tom never let a simple thing like that hold him back. He brashly called up the Chronic Respiratory Disease Control program and talked Dr. Roberts into funding such a meeting. Tom was able to convince some of the top clinicians and researchers to present at this meeting. It was an awesome achievement for an Assistant Professor of Medicine. I remember sorting the abstracts for the meeting spread all over the floor one evening in March. This conference started Tom's love for the Aspen Lung Conference. He worked tirelessly to raise funds to keep the conference going and then to start the endowment for it. His colleagues appreciated his dedication to the meeting and named the conference after him in 1989. The conference is now in the 53rd year of continuous meeting. His former secretary is the conference organizer. Aspen Lung Conference web site is www.uchsc.edu/pulmonary/aspen .

Tom was interested in Primary Care. In medical school he thought he would become a family physician. Events changed his mind and he chose pulmonary medicine. But he knew that most patients are cared for by primary care doctors. He never turned down an invitation to speak at a primary care doctors meeting. He organized education meetings for primary care for many organizations and also under the auspices of the NLHEP. He and his fishing buddies wrote a series of educational books for primary care doctors called Frontline Advice books. These were published by the Snowdrift Pulmonary Conference Inc. The topics include *Frontline Treatment of COPD 1ˢᵗ and 2ⁿᵈ editions*; *Frontline Treatment of Asthma*; *Frontline Treatment of Common Respiratory Infections, Frontline Treatment of Venous Thromboembolism*; *Frontline Assessment of Common Pulmonary Presentations*; *Frontline Assessment of Lung Cancer and Occupational Pulmonary Diseases*; *Frontline Pulmonary Procedures and Interventions*; *Frontline Treatment of Dyspnea*; and *Frontline Line Treatment of Cardiopulmonary Topics: Dyspnea*. The *Frontline* series of books, in particular, *Frontline Advice for COPD Patients*, can be downloaded for free from Dr. Petty's web site. Most of the books were written in a fishing camp in the Northwest Territories of Canada. Tom enjoyed combining his love of medicine with his great hobby of fishing.

Tom and his fishing buddies wrote one book for patients in this series *Frontline Advice for COPD Patients*. These free books were widely distributed by the Boehringer Ingelheim Company. The authors of the book included many of his former pulmonary fellow trainees. By the time they wrote the book these physicians had years of practice in academia and private practice. He co-edited the patient book with Dr. James T. Good, Jr. Jim later became Tom's personal physician after the third of his four heart surgeries. The other author contributors for the patient book were Drs. David D. Collins, Dennis E. Doherty, J. Roy Duke, Leonard D. Hudson, Thomas M. Hyers, Michael D. Iseman, Donald R. Rollins, and Charles H. Scoggin. This book and some of the others can be downloaded at Dr. Petty's web site or you may be able to find some used copies at Amazon.com. Last summer some of the original authors talked with Tom about bringing the *Frontline Advice for COPD Patients* book up-to-date. The book was published in 2002 and there have been considerable advances since then. They may take on this task in the future.

Tom was interested in the history of medicine especially the history of the pulmonary specialty. In 2000 he began to film important leaders in pulmonary medicine for what would become a classic DVD. The timing was good. Several of the leaders he was able to capture on film died before the film was released in 2001. Tom wanted to establish a documentary of physicians who made significant contributions to the field of respiratory medicine. He hoped this would give young physicians a connection to the work of their medical forefathers. In the film he traced the beginnings of blood gases and spirometry. At the Osler library in Montreal, where he was able to have access to rare manuscripts with ancient reports of lung disease, he was assisted by Dr. Jacques Danssereau. This video was widely disseminated by Boehringer Ingelheim in 2001 to 2003.

When Tom was working he was very intense. He was extremely devoted to his patients and their care. The fellows could call him night or day for consultation. He loved being a doctor. His famous saying was "patients come first." After patient care, then the research could follow. If research was of primary interest then the physician was not so much a doctor but more interested in science. He never thought of patients as subjects. Patient care was a privilege which he tried to instill in all who worked with him.

The fun side of Dr. Tom came out during conferences away from the hospital and especially during fishing trips. He enjoyed planning for fishing trips almost as much as going on the fishing excursion. He said the fun was 25% planning for fishing, 50% fishing, and the other 25% remembering the trip and looking at the pictures. We have peppered this book with some fishing quotations and some great pictures of Tom, the fisherman.

He left this world on December 12, 2009, knowing he was loved by many.

THOMAS L. PETTY, M.D.

December 24, 1932 – December 12, 2009

Thomas L. Petty, M.D., a pulmonologist, was Professor of Medicine at the University of Colorado Health Sciences Center in Denver, Rush-Presbyterian-St. Luke's Medical Center in Chicago, and Emeritus Professor of Medicine at National Jewish Health. He was previously head of the Division of Pulmonary Sciences at the University of Colorado and Director of the Fellowship Training Program. He was most recently Director of the HealthONE Center for Health Sciences Education.

Dr. Petty was organizer and founding President of the Association of Pulmonary Program Directors (APD) and has served as President of the American College of Chest Physicians. He was a former member of the Board of Governors of the American Board of Internal Medicine. Dr. Petty was the founding Chairman of the National Lung Health Education Program (NLHEP).

Dr. Petty received many honors and awards, too numerous to name here. The first such award came at his graduation from University of Colorado School of Medicine when he was given the Gold Headed Cane Award for Top Graduating Student. In 1986 Dr. Petty was given the University of Colorado Silver and Gold Award for Excellence. Dr. Petty received the Distinguished Service Award of the American Thoracic Society (1995), was elected to the Colorado Pulmonary Physicians Hall of Fame (1995), and received the Annual Award for Excellence by the American Association for Respiratory and Cardiovascular Rehabilitation (1995). He was elected to Master Fellow of the American College of Chest Physicians (1995), the fifth such award given by the ACCP in its 63-year history. He also received the Master Award of the American College of Physicians in 1996. He was awarded Fellowship in the American Association for Respiratory Care in 1999. He became Senior Fellow of the Lovelace Respiratory Research Institute in 2002. The American Association for Respiratory Care presented Dr. Petty with the Jimmy A. Young Award in 2003 and the Dr. Charles Hudson Award in 2004.

In October 2007, to honor Dr. Petty's many accomplishments in the area of respiratory medicine, The CHEST Foundation of the American College of Chest Physicians established the Thomas L. Petty, MD, Master FCCP Endowment in Lung Research. This endowment fund will support, in perpetuity, research for lung diseases, including chronic obstructive pulmonary disease (COPD), and other activities related to the improvement in care for patients with COPD and other chronic lung diseases.

Dr. Petty was founder of a quarterly newsletter, *Lung Cancer Frontiers*, and was the Editor from its inception through 2007. This newsletter is now sponsored by National Jewish Health.

Dr. Petty was an international authority on respiratory disease. He published over 800 articles in journals, including the *Journal of the American Medical Association, Chest, Annals of Internal Medicine, American Journal of Medicine, Archives of Internal Medicine, and American Journal of Respiratory & Critical Care Medicine*. He authored or was editor of 45 books or editions.

In addition to being a prolific writer, Dr. Petty was also an accomplished editor as demonstrated by the following prestigious editorial board memberships and/or appointments:

CHEST (Editor Section on Respiratory Therapy)

CHEST (Senior Editor)

RESPIRATORY CARE (Associate Editor)

HEART AND LUNG

CRITICAL CARE MEDICINE

THE WESTERN JOURNAL OF MEDICINE

SEMINARS IN RESPIRATORY AND CRITICAL CARE MEDICINE (Co-Editor-in-Chief)

MODERN MEDICINE

ARCHIVES OF INTERNAL MEDICINE

AMERICAN REVIEW OF RESPIRATORY DISEASES (Associate Editor)

IM - INTERNAL MEDICINE

RESPIRATORY MANAGEMENT (Chairman, Editorial Board)

RT (Chairman, Editorial Board)

CONTEMPORARY INTERNAL MEDICINE

RESPIRATORY EXCHANGE (Chairman, Editorial Board)

EMPHYSEMA/COPD: THE JOURNAL OF PATIENT CENTERED CARE (Honorary Chairman)

POSTGRADUATE MEDICINE

CURRENT OPINION IN PULMONARY MEDICINE

Of his many endeavors, the Thomas L. Petty Aspen Lung Conference, named after him in 1991, remained a major interest of his (web site: www.uchsc.edu/pulmonary/aspen). In addition, the newly formed TLP Moving Mountains which gave him much satisfaction to see the Colorado COPD patients and therapists offering additional programs for COPD patients (web site: www.copdconnectco.org) .

Commentary from Dr. Bernard Levine

Dr. Bernard Levine practices Pulmonary and Internal Medicine in Phoenix, Arizona. Dr. Levine graduated with an MD 51 years ago and took his pulmonary training under Dr. Petty at the University of Colorado.

Tom Petty invented pulmonary medicine as we know it today. When he started work as an assistant professor in the early 1960s, respiratory care was in its infancy. COPD was a disorder that no one wanted to talk about or treat, and oxygen was a poorly understood, inappropriately used medication. Tom Petty, a great educator and communicator, made the world aware of the importance of these disorders and their treatment. He taught us all: physicians, government agencies, and patients. And he taught us, his pulmonary fellows, to teach. Tom Petty, a superb physician, worked constantly to improve the well being of his own patients, and all patients. To those of us fortunate enough to have worked with him, he was a constant guide, a continuing inspiration, and a true friend.

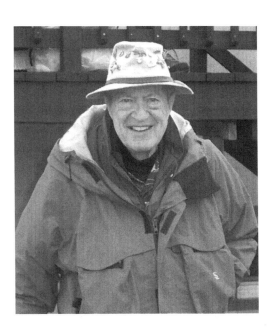

Commentary from Peter Hansen

Xolair Summit Sales Manager

One fine day, when the fishing group was up at Great Slave Lake, Tom turns to me and says, "Lets get a few beers and fish together today, it would be fun". So I proceeded to gather a few beers, which Tom commented that the beers I had looked to be enough for him but what would I be drinking, so we doubled the number of cans and off we went with our guide AJ. All the others in our group took off to the big waters of the Great Slave while we made a very short journey to our new found secret and unknown fishing spot.

Well we rigged up our fly rods and got to fishing. For quite a while nothing was happening nor were the fish biting and we both knew the unspoken rule of you needing to catch a fish first, then you can have your first beer of the day and Tom and I both were getting a bit thirsty and looking forward to "wetting our whistle".

As I was in the back of the boat with AJ we began to talk about his native spirits and traditions and we decided that I needed to provide an offering to the native spirits, so with that AJ gave me a cigarette and about the same moment that AJ gave me that cigarette Tom turned around and saw me with that cigarette and YOU SHOULD HAVE SEEN THE LOOK IN HIS EYES !!! First he starts what was I doing with that cigarette and surely I had no intention of actually smoking it.....Well I assured Tom that I was not but that AJ and I had agreed that I needed to make an offering to the native spirit of great fishing. So I gently opened up the cigarette and sprinkled the tobacco into the water right where we were fishing.....Guess what in a couple of moments.....WHAM a huge Lake Trout got on my fly and we fought for a while until he was landed and released. Tom said nice fish, but to hell with the tobacco idea.....then on very next cast WHAM another huge Lake Trout on the fly which I landed and released.

All of sudden Tom said "Give me one of those damned cigarettes so I can start catching fish" and guess what he did !!! The moral of the story which Tom and I both decided was not to mess with the Spirits of Fishing and if they want a cigarette then give it to them !!!

WITH LOVE FROM PETER

Foreword

Louise Nett

The inspiration for this book came from Dr. Thomas L. Petty, a pulmonary physician, a Professor of Medicine, a researcher, a role model, a great and loyal friend, a fisherman, an organizer, a story teller, a world traveler and teacher, and a doctor who loved patients.

Tom wrote several books for patients. The forerunner of this one, *Adventures of an Oxy-Phile*, is now out of print but it is available on his website. In his last years Tom was challenged with a number of health issues, but continued to write and consult despite all these illnesses. He decided to author this book in August of 2009 after a reprieve and a feeling of well-being gave him the hope he could write one more book for patients. He was blessed to see most of the chapters before his death. Finishing the book fell to Louise Nett, his colleague and friend of 44 years, and his secretary, Kay Bowen, with the assistance of Debbie Bunch, Bob McCoy, and with the help of book designer, Don Eastburn.

Thomas L. Petty, MD graduated from the University of Colorado Medical School in 1958. He interned in Philadelphia and did a year of residency in Michigan before returning to Denver in 1960, where he spent the rest of his life. He rose through the academic ranks to become a full Professor of Medicine at the University of Colorado and also had the rank of Professor of Medicine at Rush/Presbyterian in Chicago, and Emeritus Professor of Medicine at National Jewish Health. Tom was active in medicine until his death December 12, 2009.

Tom was a young assistant professor of medicine at the University of Colorado when I (LN) met him. He had a promise from Dr. Gordon Meiklejohn, the Chairman of the Department of Medicine, that he would have a laboratory in the new University of Colorado hospital when it opened at the end of the month (Feb 1965). He also had a salary for a full time nurse and a half time blood gas technician, Susie Tyler. I was the nurse. Tom called this new lab the Respiratory Care Laboratory. He came back from a trip to the Karolinska Institute in Stockholm Sweden, where they had blood gas analysis right next to the critical care patients. I must admit when he told me that the lab would measure the gases in the blood, I was a bit perplexed. I knew nothing about measuring oxygen and carbon dioxide (ABGs) in the blood. He said not to worry as we would all learn together.

Tom and his surgical partner, Dr. David Ashbaugh, the pulmonary fellows and I started patient care rounds at 7:30AM (not 7:31AM). Dr. Tom was a stickler for punctuality. The pulmonary team consisted of the pulmonary fellows in training….. Dr. Bernard Levine, Dr. Boyd Bigelow, and Dr. Neil Goldberg. It was an adventure. Everything was new to us. Actually what we were doing was new to just about everybody in the US. Cardiac care units were catching on but pulmonary intensive care units lagged behind.

We were doing a study of COPD patients on the research unit at the same time as starting the critical care unit. Patients were admitted for a month of disease stabilization. Measurements were taken of their activity level and medical status during this time. The next month, patients received continuous oxygen. Again regular measurements were taken. It was amazing to see the improvement in exercise and feeling of well-being during the month on oxygen. We were one of the first sites that received the new Linde oxygen walker. It was a light-weight canister of liquid oxygen that made portable oxygen a possibility. This was the start of our pulmonary rehabilitation program which included continuous home oxygen therapy. We learned very quickly that it was important to stop the "revolving door" of COPD patients. We knew we had to improve their care at home or they would be back in the hospital in a short time. We started educating COPD patients in self management of medications, oxygen therapy, and an exercise program.

At the American Thoracic Society meeting in May and the 8th Aspen Lung Conference in June of 1965, the fellows presented papers on the improvement these patients exhibited on oxygen therapy. There was some criticism since the prevailing concept was that patients would retain carbon dioxide and go into coma if given oxygen. This did not turn out to be the case and LTOT was off and running. The chief of the Chronic Disease program in Washington DC was present for the meeting in Aspen. He asked Tom to come to their department to present this new data. Tom came back with a new grant to study the rehabilitation of COPD patients (including the use of oxygen).

Following the good results with treatment for COPD patients and the use of long term oxygen therapy, Tom was asked to lecture at many US meetings. As they say he "had bag and will travel" to teach about modern day respiratory care. He started publishing research papers and books about respiratory care. His first book for physicians was titled *Intensive and Rehabilitative Respiratory Care* published in 1971. Then came the requests to travel abroad to teach these new concepts. And travel he did to South America, Europe, the Far East, and Australia. Probably the country he had most impact on regarding oxygen therapy was Japan, where he made many trips to speak to physicians, nurses, and patients. Dr. Shiro Kira of Juntendo University School of Medicine and Dr. Petty co-authored a book Progress in Domiciliary Respiratory Care following the meeting in Tokyo in 1993 on the same topic. Presenters from all over Europe and from the Far East presented papers on current status of oxygen and home care.

Dr. Petty received many honors and awards in his lifetime. The patients and caregivers of Colorado honored him in October 2009 by calling the patient education meeting after him. The Thomas L. Petty Moving Mountains Conference is a meeting held in Denver, Colorado every fall. Many directors of Respiratory Rehabilitation Programs, medical supply vendors, and most of all patients meet for months to plan the annual program. The content varies from year to year with the express purpose of teaching chronic lung patients about the newest and latest information of interest to them. He felt this honor was the best thank you that he could receive for his years of dedication to patients and caregivers who knew him.

— *Louise Nett*

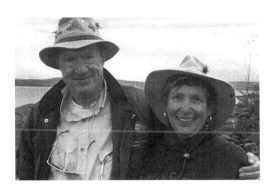

ADVENTURES OF AN OXY-PHILE$_2$

*By Thomas L. Petty, M.D. with Robert McCoy, B.S., RRT, FAARC,
Louise M. Nett, RN, RRT, & Kay Bowen*

*Editorial Assistants: Debbie Bunch, BA and Diane B. Seebass, BA, MA
Reviewers: Keene Jorgensen, Ron Peterson, Joe Walsh and Authors*

*"They say you forget your troubles on a trout stream, but that's not quite it.
What happens is that you begin to see where your troubles fit into the grand
scheme of things, and suddenly they're just not such a big deal anymore."*
— John Gierach —

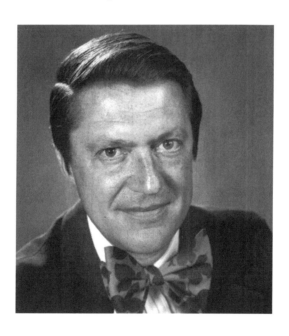

Preface to Second Edition

Thomas L. Petty, M.D.

2009

Nearly six years have passed since the writing of the first edition. During that period of time, there have been immense advances in oxygen technology. There are unfortunate and restrictive controls on oxygen reimbursement. There is an overwhelming need for new science to determine whether or not patients with mild to moderate hypoxemia need supplemental oxygen. These studies are a long way off. Many patients have unanswered questions about oxygen therapy. I have answered some of these questions appearing in the popular American Association For Respiratory Care column *"Ask Dr. Tom"* (web site: www.yourlunghealth.org). A second edition of *Adventures of an Oxy-Phile* was deemed necessary due to the immense experience accumulated in the past six years.

This book is written for all Oxy-Philes, their caregivers, and respiratory therapists. It is particularly valuable for the motivation of people who want to continue to pursue life and happiness by virtue of long term oxygen therapy (LTOT).

PREFACE TO FIRST EDITION*
Thomas L. Petty, M.D. - 2003

In 1965, we began our original scientific studies in long term home oxygen therapy. This has become known as LTOT. The true adventure began on one snowy February day in 1965. Louise M. Nett, a nurse and now a respiratory therapist, and I (TLP) went to a dark basement where we

*The first edition of *Adventures of an Oxy-Phile* is a free download at http://drtompetty.org.

were told to go find and fill some new oxygen equipment. This was the original Linde Walker & Reservoir prototype system that was shipped from New York to my mentor, the late Roger S. Mitchell. Roger assigned us to unpack the devices, set them up, and get them to work.

After reading the instructions, we carefully placed the canister upside down over the filling port of the reservoir to make a connection. A loud hissing sound happened and scared us, so we backed out of the room. This was the normal sound of liquid oxygen being transferred to the ambulatory canister which could be carried by the patient. When the hissing stopped, we disconnected the walking device and pressed the start button that was marked 2L. We were pleased and surprised to hear oxygen flowing. We attached tubing to nasal prongs and breathed the oxygen for a few minutes. Subsequently we completed our first pilot studies with six very hypoxic patients. We reported our preliminary results at the 8th Aspen Emphysema Conference in June 1965. Many in academia were stunned by our brazen behavior: giving oxygen to COPD cripples! We were warned by some of the senior doctors from New York that "everyone knows" it is dangerous to give oxygen to COPD patients because of the risk of severe carbon dioxide buildup. We never believed this was dangerous and already had done arterial blood gases that demonstrated that controlled low flow oxygen not only corrected the deficit, but did not result in carbon dioxide buildup.

Over the years that followed, our group and others established the scientific basis for oxygen therapy with an emphasis on ambulatory oxygen. We wrote our original articles on LTOT in the late 1960s. In the mid 1970s we organized and supervised the conduct of the Nocturnal Oxygen Therapy Trial (NOTT), which set the scientific basis for oxygen as it is used today in patients with oxygen deficits due to COPD and related disorders. The results of the NOTT were published in 1980. We have also been involved in the development of new oxygen technologies from the very beginning right up to the present time. Thus the Denver studies and more extensive multicenter trials gradually established the scientific basis for long term oxygen therapy (LTOT). Today LTOT is available in all modernized societies, but is little used in large areas of the world. Ambulatory oxygen using modern low weight devices is established as the standard of care.

Now, following my fourth open-heart surgery and severe pulmonary hypertension, I (TLP) am amongst the ranks of the LTOT users. Thus I have a full perspective about oxygen, from its scientific origins to its present day applications. In the final analysis, we are all "oxy-philes." That is, we literally love oxygen. Oxygen allows for the energy possessed in all of the cells, tissues, and organs of our body. Oxygen allows us to live and pursue life to its fullest. This book is written for and by patients who have learned to adapt to the need for supplemented oxygen. We authors hope it will serve thousands of patients and their families, as well as other students of oxygen.

"There is something in fishing that tends to produce a gentleness of spirit and a pure sincerity of mind."
— Washington Irving —

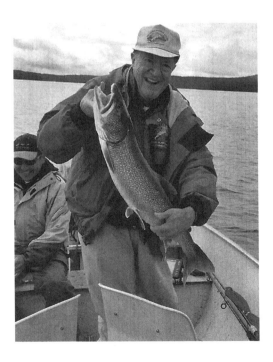

""What are more delightful than one's emotions when approaching
a trout stream for the initial cast?"
— T. Nash Buckingham —

Chapter 1

The Need for Oxygen

Thomas L. Petty, M.D.

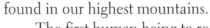

Every cell of the body needs oxygen for high energy production. Oxygen is at the end of a complex energy electron transfer chain that allows the "wheels" of energy production to function smoothly. Thus oxygen and the energy it produces enable the body to maintain the integrity of the cells that comprise our tissues and organs. Without oxygen, these cells quickly die or, at least, are damaged until a repair process can take place. Current evidence indicates that early mild to moderate damage to the cells of the lung may be repaired by continuous oxygen use at rest and exercise.

Humans can adapt to high altitude and, indeed, small communities can be sustained in the Peruvian Andes as high as 17,000 feet, where the oxygen saturation is about 75-80% due to compensations. Even though a few mountain climbers have ascended to higher elevations and have climbed Mount Everest, the highest place on earth, without oxygen, man cannot survive a sustained oxygen deficit equivalent to that found in our highest mountains.

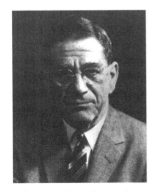

The first human being to receive oxygen in a hospital was a young man with severe bacterial pneumonia in York Hospital in 1885. Dr. George Holtzapple gave oxygen produced by chemicals, similar to what Joseph Priestley, the discoverer of oxygen had done about 100 years earlier. The young man survived. Soon after that humble beginning, oxygen tents were pioneered in the treatment of life-threatening pneumonia. The late Alvan Barach of New York invented the first

Alvan L. Barach

practical oxygen tent in 1920 and reported widely on his experience to the scientific and lay press.

Over the years industry has developed an impressive array of new oxygen technologies. These began with high pressure compressed gas cylinders, which were the standard for hospital and home use until the early 1960s. Next came liquid portable oxygen, which is an inexpensive and practical oxygen supply for both hospitals and the home. The advent of the liquid oxygen "walker" was a technological breakthrough first studied in 1965 and later more extensively evaluated by the Denver group. Later the Nocturnal Oxygen Therapy Trial (NOTT) of the 1970s published in 1980 created a sound scientific basis for LTOT ambulatory oxygen use being superior to stationary oxygen. This evolving research has led to evolutionary changes that have improved liquid oxygen technology to the point that very practical modern ambulatory oxygen systems weighing approximately four pounds are now in common use.

Oxygen concentrators were introduced in the 1970s. Concentrators separate the oxygen from the nitrogen and other inert gases in the air. Today they are the most practical and efficient sources for stationary oxygen used in the home. But being homebound is not the goal of an Oxy-Phile. Low weight concentrators providing a sufficient output and weighing approximately 10 pounds are suitable for most ambulatory activities. Only intermittent flow delivery is provided by the portable devices.

Low weight, high pressure compressed oxygen in tanks also of low weight, can be used effectively with ambulation and full activities of daily living but they lack the convenience and efficiency of liquid portable systems and are not less costly if used in full activities of daily living.

A new battery-powered or electricity-powered oxygen concentrator useful in travel and for limited portability arrived in the market over the last few years. It is the truly portable concentrator that provides continuous flow up to 3L per minute. Continuous flow is important in nighttime mouth breathing. More details about oxygen, oxygen technologies, oxygen prescribing, and related matters can be found in Chapter 4.

This book is not about just the science and technology of oxygen; it is about the people who need oxygen and benefit from it.

"Fishing is the chance to wash one's soul with pure air, with the rush of the brook, or with the shimmer of the sun on blue water.."

— Herbert Hoover —

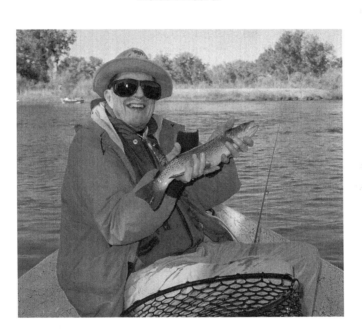

Chapter 2

Early Experiences as an Oxy-Phile

Thomas L. Petty, M.D

Following our original work with oxygen, which began in 1965, and our original report, we became interested in certain personal side benefits of oxygen. In 1968, I first took a 9-pound "Linde Walker" on a hike up to a high mountain lake where I love to fish for trout. "How easy it was to walk at 12,000 feet," I thought to myself, having climbed these same mountains many times before with much more shortness of breath and effort than I experienced with the portable oxygen system.

Later I took the growing Division of Pulmonary Medicine at the University of Colorado Hospital on our first annual hike, which we initiated in August 1972. My outfit *(photo top right)*, contains a liquid oxygen device, a leather bottle filled with wine, and my fishing rod and creel. It was easy to walk the ascending four miles from "The Fourth of July campground" at 7,000 feet to 12,000 feet at Dorothy Lake near the Continental Divide with the assistance of lightweight oxygen.

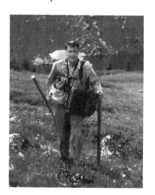

My climbing outfit (1972)

In 1984 I tested out a prototype of a demand control system (oxygen conserving device), a forerunner of pulse delivery technology used in new ambulatory devices, on another outing of the division as we climbed up to Diamond Lake from the same campground at nearly 11,000 feet in 1984. The photo *(bottom right)* is a candid picture of a

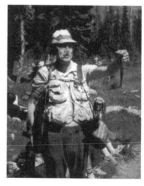

Diamond Lake, 11,000 ft.

small cutthroat native trout in the foreground caught on a dry fly (#16 Adams.) Some of the fellows and faculty are seen in the background.

These early experiences gave me an inkling about what it is like to "wear oxygen." I saw considerable advantages from using lightweight oxygen at the high altitudes frequently experienced in the Rocky Mountains, 9000-14,000 feet above sea level. This modern experience in a simple way is reminiscent of how mountaineers used oxygen while attempting to climb the highest peak in the world, Mount Everest. In 1924 George Mallory was seen disappearing into the clouds at approximately 28,000 feet, carrying oxygen, in a failed struggle to reach the summit. He was never seen again. Sir Edmond Hillary and his loyal guide, Tensing, climbed Everest in 1953 with the assistance of oxygen. Subsequently, Everest has been climbed both with and without oxygen, but with great difficulty and the possibility of at least subtle degrees of brain damage. The human body simply cannot survive below a certain level of oxygen tension and even moments on top of Mount Everest with an oxygen saturation of about 45% begin to take their toll.

Now that I am a regular oxygen user because of a complex set of problems following my fourth open-heart surgery and reversible renal failure which was a result of antibiotics, I am looking at oxygen from "the other end of the stethoscope."[1]

Although my early research and personal experiences continue to serve me well, we need new and expanded ideas, more clinical research, and even better technologies to make greater progress. I still fish, but mostly from shore in small lakes or from a boat. The photo *(page 10)* shows a 25" Rainbow caught on the Big Horn River with Guide Mark Stroda of Ft. Smith, Montana. The river is at 2000 feet, which explains why I am not using oxygen while seated in the boat. The liquid portable system (not seen) is needed for me to be able to walk to the parking lot, which is 250 yards up a steep hill. I simply could not do this without oxygen.

The past nearly 40 years have provided marvelous evolution in the treatment for advanced stages of COPD and related disorders with oxygen, which is best provided by lightweight ambulatory systems, most commonly ultra lightweight liquid oxygen containers; e.g., Helios, Spirit 300, and others. There will be even lighter oxygen devices for the patient to wear in the near future.

1 *From Both Ends of the Stethoscope*, written by Thomas L. Petty, M.D., ©2008, or www.drtompetty.org

"More than half the intense enjoyment of fly-fishing is derived from the beautiful surroundings, the satisfaction felt from being in the open air, the new lease of life secured thereby, and the many, many pleasant recollections of all one has seen, heard and done."

— Charles F. Orvis —

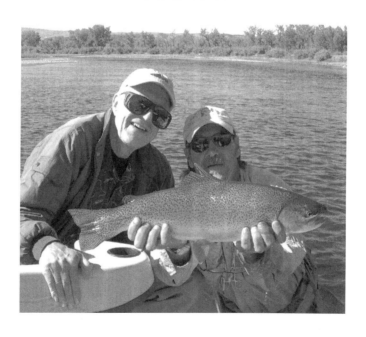

Chapter 3

Common Questions
Asked by Patients*

Thomas L. Petty, MD

Do I really need oxygen?

The answer to this question for most patients is "yes." Everyone needs an oxygen supply because oxygen is key to the high energy production system of the body. Measurements are made by your physician to indicate the level of oxygenation accomplished in your blood. Normally it should be more than 88% saturated; that is, the blood should carry a minimum of 88% of the oxygen under perfect conditions. This is also known as an oxygen tension of 55 mm. Often the oxygen is needed if there has been a recent hospitalization for heart failure. This oxygen allows the heart and lungs to adequately support circulation in a life-threatening situation.

What will my friends think?

As is the case with most medical equipment used by patients, your family and friends will think that you are doing good things to improve your quality and length of life by using oxygen. You should consider it "cool" — and the right thing to do.

Will I get hooked on oxygen?

The answer to this question is, of course you will, since everyone is hooked on oxygen. But you will not get hooked on oxygen the same way someone gets hooked on a narcotic. It is easy to discontinue the use of oxygen if your pulmonary or cardiac disease improves adequately.

---

* Editor's Note (LN): Dr. Petty answered these questions before his death in December of 2009.

Do I need a personal oximeter?

The personal oximeter industry has provided a simple, one-ounce device that can be attached to the fingertip. This device shows the pulse of the arterial oxygenated blood that has already received oxygen from the lungs. The oximeter should be used as a personal dosing instrument, with the patient not only allowed, but encouraged, to make changes in liter flow depending on oxygen needs that may be encountered with exercise, ascent to altitude, or change in medical condition. Too many doctors, nurses, and respiratory therapists want to be the "controller" when it comes to the use of oxygen. Today, simple home oximeters cost less than $100. These are very reliable and serviceable, and should be used by all patients on long term oxygen therapy (LTOT).

How many people use oxygen and how are they receiving it?

Presently there are approximately 1.4 million Americans who receive oxygen by all systems, including liquid, gaseous, and concentrators. Concentrators are becoming more popular since more and more of them are becoming lightweight (ten pounds or less). Heavyweight concentrators are used only in the home. New units weighing in at 17 pounds can also deliver continuous or intermittent oxygen flow and use AC house current or batteries. This makes them ideal for both travel and home use. They use low energy and are pleasantly quiet.*

About 400,000 patients receive liquid portable oxygen by various systems in the United States. There are a growing number of systems that will add to our armamentarium in the use of truly wearable oxygen in the future. Liquid oxygen is widely used in Italy, but otherwise only sparsely used throughout the rest of the industrialized world.

What is transtracheal oxygen?

Transtracheal oxygen (TTO) is a method of delivering oxygen directly into the trachea, with a pre-established portal that requires a minor surgical procedure. This device not only increases the efficiency of oxygen, but also has the advantage of concealing oxygen use in patients who are embarrassed

---

* Editorial Note (LN): Today it is believed that there are 2,000,000 Americans who receive supplemental oxygen.

about their use of oxygen. It should be used in more and more patients because recent research shows it tends to improve shortness of breath. Today there are proposals for more oxygen studies to help establish LTOT. We need more studies on the benefit of TTO as well. *(See photo bottom left.)* Chapter 7 features more details on TTO.

Are there any other devices to help conceal oxygen use?

A cosmetic improvement can also be made via the Oxy-Frames *(see image bottom right.)* This is a simply modified cannulae attached to a pair of eyeglasses. Many patients find it comfortable and pleasant to wear.

What are the Oxygen Consensus Conferences and how have they impacted LTOT?

Six Oxygen Consensus Conferences have been organized by the Denver Group and have been held in Denver and Washington, D.C. Summaries of the proceedings can be found on the web at http://www.ltotnet.org/resources.html. Results from these conferences have helped to inform both the opportunities and challenges in the LTOT arena over the past 20 years.

Is there any new research going on in LTOT?

There are proposed new studies to evaluate whether oxygen is useful

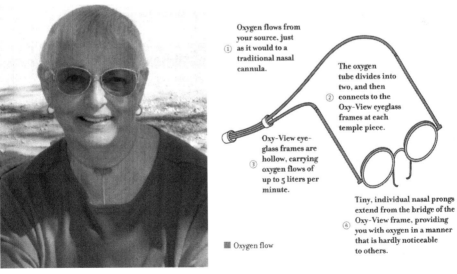

Transtracheal oxygen user (TTO)   Oxy-Frames

in improving quality and length of life in patients with only mild degrees of hypoxemia; for example, those with oxygen tensions higher than 55 mm and saturations higher than 88%. Such a study is hard to organize and recruit and it will probably be a decade before one is completed. We would also like to see the inclusion of transtracheal oxygen in new oxygen therapy trials. See Chapter 20.

When and whether such studies will ever be accomplished, however, remains to be seen. It is a fact that no new controlled clinical science has been contributed to LTOT since the completion of the NOTT study and the British MRC studies in the late 1970s, both of which were published in 1980.

What advancements do you see in LTOT going forward?

In the future, oxygen use must be more patient friendly. There are new technologies to be brought to bear that will develop oxygen without either the necessity of creating a liquid phase or using a molecular sieve. We are depending on industry to develop newer equipment that is easier to use and less costly. It is essential that third party payers understand the value of oxygen for patients as well, so that these new technologies will actually be produced and reimbursed.

What's the take home message from this book?

It is apparent from the contents of this book that an immense amount of progress has been made in the use of LTOT in COPD and related disorders where hypoxemia — a true deficit in the arterial oxygenated blood — is present. Oxygen improves both the length and quality of life. Improved technology has made oxygen more accessible, and ambulatory patients may be able to lead more independent and productive lives with today's technology.

*"All the romance of trout fishing exists in the mind of the angler
and is in no way shared by the fish."*

— Harold F. Blaisdell —

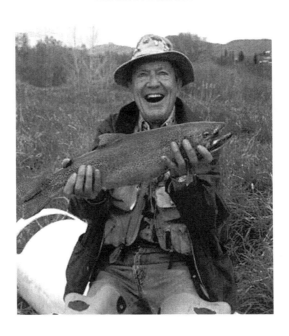

Chapter 4

OXYGEN

Reprinted from the First Edition of Adventures

Thomas L. Petty, M.D.

Oxygen is the most common element in the earth's crust. Thus, it is obviously part of God's plan. Most oxygen, however, exists in the form of oxygen involved in mineral and rocks. The oxygen that we breathe does not come from this source. It comes from the process of photosynthesis, which is the conversion of carbon dioxide to oxygen that only plants can do. The vast majority of photosynthesis occurs in algae in the sea. Carbon dioxide originally came from the atmosphere, which probably resulted from "the big bang." In any case, carbon dioxide and photosynthesis create oxygen.

Joseph Priestly, a Unitarian minister, first isolated oxygen from chemicals and breathed (along with two mice) this mixture in 1774 . "Who knows, but in that time this pure air (Priestly's word for oxygen) would become a fashionable article of luxury." How prophetic. Yet oxygen is not a luxury; it is a necessity of life. Priestly's American home in the borough of Northhumberland, Pennsylvania, at the branch of the Susquehanna River, is preserved as a museum and should be visited by all Oxy-Philes.

As all energy on earth can be traced to the sun's energy, it is appropriate to trace the evolution of oxygen to the sun because the earth's original oxygen was most likely formed by the photo-dissociation of water by ultraviolet light from the sun. The amount of oxygen produced this way was small and probably of the order of magnitude of about one-thousandth the oxygen concentration presently in our atmosphere. In fact, the amount of oxygen was probably fixed until the development of life itself because it is a living process, photosynthesis that creates most of the oxygen in the atmosphere. Photosynthesis began approximately a billion years ago when early traces of algae were formed from water, carbon dioxide, and ammonia that were available in the primordial sea that bathed most of this planet. First came a series of more complex organic compounds and finally the first primitive photosynthesis cells that were crucial to the evolution of all life. Briefly the process of photosynthesis is the reaction of:

CO_2 + H_2 + UV + chlorophyll = O_2 + by-products.

At this point in the evolution of the earth, the atmospheric oxygen concentration increased rapidly to a new order of magnitude. The final concentration became stabilized by the fact that the increased production of oxygen encouraged respiration and the consumption of oxygen, which in turn reduced the amount of oxygen available. Thus, by about a half a billion years ago there was very active photosynthetic life and the evolution of multicellular organisms in water. However, it took many millions of years for enough ozone to be generated from oxygen to be released into the atmosphere, which in turn would screen out the ultraviolet light to a sufficient degree to permit life to exist on land. These steps in the evolution of oxygen are intimately intertwined with the evolution of life itself and the transition of life from sea to land. Once an atmospheric "steady state," meaning a balance between production and consumption of oxygen, was achieved, terrestrial life and further evolution became possible.

The concentration of oxygen in the air is 20.9%; and this concentration has remained constant during the evolution of higher forms of life, including man. Somewhere in this evolution, the oxidative enzymes developed together with the mitochondria that are necessary factors to maintain the cellular integrity and function of aerobic organisms. Mitochondria are dedicated to energy production. Most of the oxygen that reaches the mitochondria is "handled" in the production of high-energy phosphate bonds (ATP). Oxygen functions as an electron acceptor and allows energy to be produced by electron transfer from hydrogen activation from foodstuffs. Thus, living systems made of matter must be driven by energy; and oxygen is essential in this energy cascade! Oxygen is also used by enzymes called oxygenases that are necessary in the development of neurotransmitters that control the functional integrity of the intact organism. Thus, oxygen, which is one of the most common elements in the earth's crust (as water or part of the matrix of minerals, but in this form unavailable for respiration) is an essential ingredient for aerobic life. Oxygen consumption is central to the process of energy development, much of which is used for the maintenance of cellular and, thus, tissue integrity as well as the functional control of integrated organ systems. Without this, there could be no life as we understand it.

So much for the history of the evolution of oxygen — a colorless, odorless, tasteless gas upon which we depend so absolutely and completely. Yet oxygen is essentially taken for granted unless it becomes in short supply!

The oxygen is breathed, thus traversing the upper and lower airways by the process of ventilation, and is then transmitted across the alveolocapillary membrane barrier by diffusion to the hemoglobin and carried to the tissues for the process of high energy metabolism in the mitochondria. The oxygen tensions (pressures available for gas movement) in each of these steps are depicted in Figure 17, based upon sea level values. The concen-

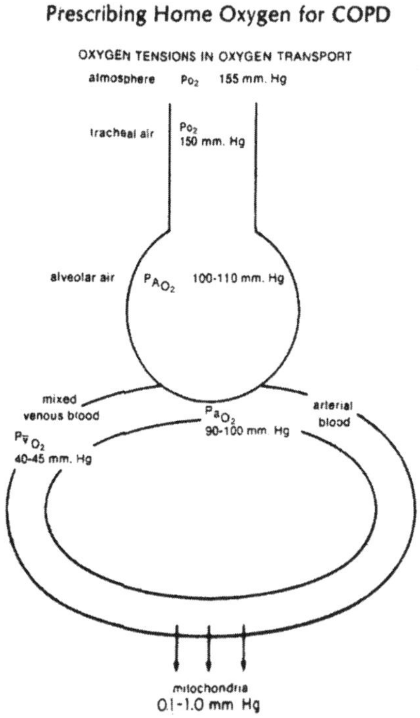

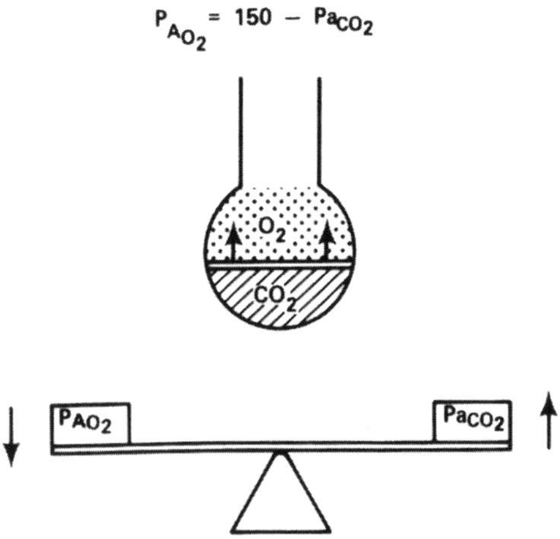

Prescribing Home Oxygen for COPD

Figure 17. Oxygen tensions in the transport of oxygen to the tissues beginning with atmospheric tension. Tracheal air oxygen tension, alveolar air oxygen tension, arterial oxygen tension, probable oxygen tension at the mitochondrial level where metabolism takes place and normal mixed venous oxygen tensions are listed.

Figure 18. Graphic representation of the reciprocal relationship between alveolar oxygen tension and CO2 tension. An assumption is made that arterial and alveolar CO2 tensions are the same, which is essentially true in health. A modified alveolar air equation makes the same assumption (top of figure).

tration of oxygen in the atmosphere, of course, is fixed at 20.9% but the amount of oxygen in the inspired air is inversely proportional to altitude in a fairly linear fashion as illustrated in Table 5.

The arterial oxygen tension in relation to altitude is not perfectly linear because of ventilatory compensations caused by the response to hypoxemia. With augmented ventilation, the alveolar and, thus, the arterial oxygen tension are slightly increased due to the reciprocal relationship between alveolar PO2 and PCO2 in the alveolar air *(Figure 18)*. This affects the resulting arterial oxygen and carbon dioxide tensions *(Table 5)*.

Also, because of the shape of the oxygen hemoglobin dissociation curve, Figure 19, a significant reduction in inspired and, thus, arterial PO2 can occur with little effect on oxygen amount (i.e., oxygen saturation). Oxygen saturation refers to the amount of oxygen carried by hemoglobin compared to the capacity for oxygen carried under ideal conditions expressed as a percent *(Figure 19)*. This is why the oxygen tension can fall from a normal of 80 to 100 at sea level to 60 to 70 at Denver with essentially no difference in the oxygen saturation of hemoglobin as dictated by the oxyhemoglobin dissociation curve.

Greater altitudes begin to stress the system; but compensations of increased cardiac output, adjustments in red cell mass with shifts in the oxyhemoglobin dissociation curve to the left to carry more oxygen, and some

Table 5: Oxygen Tensions of Various Altitudes (mm Hg) Inhabited by Man

Meters	Feet (Approx.)	Barometric Pressure	PIO2	PaO2	SaO2	PaCO2
0	0	760	149	95	98	41
1,500	5,000	630	122	67	92	38
2,500	8,000	564	108	60	89	37
3,000	10,000	523	100	53	85	36
3,600	12,000	483	91	52	83	35
4,600	15,000	412	76	44	75	31
5,500	18,000	379	69	40	71	29

fancy biochemical adjustments that will allow for the unloading of oxygen at the tissue level to be more efficiently increased (2, 3-diphosphoglycerate), allow for adaptation to high altitudes. Thus, man can exist for at least short periods at the highest reaches of our planet. Mt. Everest, for example, has been ascended recently without the aid of supplemental oxygen! This almost unbelievable feat, however, is only possible by virtue of exquisitely responsive compensatory mechanisms that include cardiac output, red cell mass, biochemical alterations of blood favoring delivery of oxygen to tissues, and probably the tolerance of a low level of oxygen, which if sustained could not support life. Figure 20 reproduces the oxyhemoglobin dissociation curve and indicates the oxygen tensions where man has lived or climbed!

When we return to the purpose of this brief monograph which is the use of oxygen in patients with COPD and related disorders i.e., "oxy-philes" — we must be constantly mindful of the fact that the individual patient with hypoxemia is not endowed with athletic compensatory mechanisms. Thus, they may suffer severe consequences of hypoxemia such as pulmonary hypertension, right heart strain, cerebral dysfunction, and possibly other organ system dysfunction at higher levels of arterial oxygenation than do normal people with these compensations. Indeed, and perhaps more importantly, the patient with COPD, usually older and less physically fit and

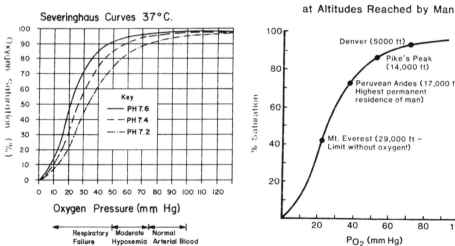

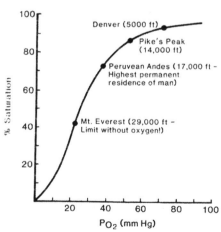

Figure 19. Classic Severinghaus oxyhemoglobin dissociation curve relating oxygen saturation to oxygen tension. Effect of pH change is indicated.

Figure 20. Oxygen saturation in relation to altitudes achieved by man.

having been exposed to many years of hypoxemia, finally succumbs to the ravages of oxygen lack. This usually occurs at a sustained arterial oxygen tension of 55 or less. It must be admitted, however, that there is considerable individual variation in a patient's ability to tolerate hypoxemia. Many normal individuals can live comfortably and productively at high altitudes, as high as 17,000 feet, in the Peruvian Mountains with oxygen tensions in the high 30s and no apparent damage. In fact, some patients with COPD and chronic levels of severe hypoxemia (e.g., PO2 40 to 50) seem to tolerate this partly anaerobic state very well for reasons that are not entirely understood. Thus, man can live in relative comfort at a barometric pressure that is reduced by nearly one-half and with what clinicians would view as alarming hypoxemia; but this is only possible by major compensatory mechanisms that are not present in most patients with advanced COPD.

This book deals with the COPD patient and others who are candidates for oxygen, and the value of oxygen therapy, particularly ambulatory oxygen; approaches to the therapy that may return the patient to a functional optimum. The focus is on oxygen therapy, which is often an important step in preserving health and functioning and preventing or forestalling premature morbidity or mortality from COPD and related disorders. It also focuses on the various evolving oxygen systems and their respective advantages in certain clinical situations.

PRESCRIBING LTOT — *Indications for LTOT*

The table below lists the commonly accepted indications for LTOT and the requirements for oxygen prescription from the Centers for Medicare and Medicaid Services (CMS), formerly known as Health Care Financing Administration (HCFA) and certain insurance plans. When daytime normoxia is present, but sleep related hypoxemia has been established by continuous nocturnal monitoring of oxygen saturation, oxygen can be prescribed during the hours of sleep when there is clinical evidence of harm from the consequences of hypoxemia, i.e., morning headaches, clinical evidence of pulmonary hypertension and erythrocytosis. Similarly, if exercise-related hypoxemia is demonstrated by pulse oximetry, ambulatory oxygen can be prescribed and is particularly appropriate if it can be demonstrated that improved exercise-tolerance results are from ambulatory oxygen therapy.

Table 5: General Prescribing Guidelines for Home Oxygen Patients with Advanced COPD

PATIENT SELECTION CRITERIA
Stable course of disease on optimum indicated medical therapy, e.g., bronchodilator, antibiotics, corticosteroids
At least two arterial blood gas determinations while breathing air for at least 20 minutes
Room air PO2 consistently 55 or less, or consistently 55 to 59 + cor pulmonale clinically diagnosed, or hematocrit 55% or greater
Normoxic patients, when less dyspnea and increased exercise tolerance are demonstrated with oxygen
OXYGEN DOSE
Continuous flow by double lumen nasal cannula
By demand system with demonstration of adequate oxygen saturation
Lowest liter flow to raise PO2 to 60 to 65 or oxygen saturation to 88% to 94%
Increase baseline liter flow by 1 liter/min. during exercise and sleep
EXPECTED OUTCOMES
There are many benefits of LTOT for patients who require it. Some of the most noted and well-documented outcomes are:
Improved tolerance of exercise and other ambulatory activities
Decreased pulmonary hypertension
Improved neuropsychiatric function
Decreased erythrocytosis and polycythemia
Reduced morbidity and mortality
Increased length of life

"Many men go fishing all of their lives without knowing that it is not fish they are after"

— Henry David Thoreau —

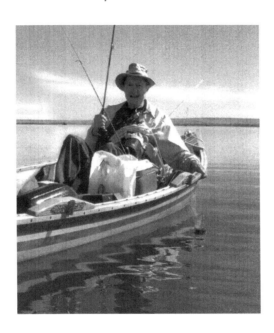

Chapter 5

Living with COPD

Gene Schwarz, MD

Perhaps the title of this chapter should be, "Accepting You Have Chronic Obstructive Pulmonary Disease, and Learning to Live With It." That was the difficult part for me. As a clinical professor of psychiatry at the University of Colorado Health Sciences Center and a former director of The Denver Institute for Psychoanalysis, I should have seen the psychological issues coming. But in many respects, I didn't.

It all started right after I turned 65 and joined the Medicare rolls. My primary care physician announced he was retiring and referred me to a young colleague, telling me I would be better off with someone who most likely would outlive me.

This young doctor was very thorough, and one of the questions he asked me was, "Do you smoke?" I said, "No." He then asked if I had ever smoked, and I could sense a bit of irritation arising in me, which I managed to ignore. I gave him a short, quick affirmative response, which seemed to propel him to delve into my smoking history.

He finally dragged out of me the fact that I had my first cigarette at age nine and my last at age 49. He thought 40 years of smoking warranted a more thorough evaluation of my pulmonary function and took me into another room where he had a portable spirometer.

The results of this simple test indicated that I had COPD. I had no symptoms of this disease and was living a healthy life, with exercise and good nutrition all while living at an altitude of 8000 feet. I could ski, ride a bike, and do moderate workouts. So I had COPD. So what?

Down the river of denial

I never told my wife or family about my visit with my new doctor, and I managed to avoid seeing him and any other doctor for the next seven years. I did not consciously decide to keep this diagnosis secret or not to go back to the doctor. It just happened. It is as if after leaving his office I left all that he told me behind.

This young man was a discerning diagnostician, but I don't think he fully appreciated the impact of being told you have a serious progressive disease. After 50 years in psychiatry, I can spot massive denial a mile away. I just couldn't see it when it was under my nose.

At age 72, I developed a fulminating pneumonia, and for the first time I can remember, I was very, very sick. I would like to say when I recovered I finally acknowledged I needed to have my pulmonary function evaluated, but it took another bout of pneumonia the following year to break through this powerful state of denial.

In retrospect, even at age 65, I had symptoms of a compromised pulmonary function that I managed to ignore. My wife tells me she also ignored the moments I had shortness of breath, and in a sense was colluding with my denial of there being something wrong going on in my body. She didn't want me to be sick, and neither did I.

You might think this is the old story of, what you don't know or won't acknowledge, won't hurt you. It's really the story of how painfully frightening it is to have something going on in your body that you can't control, and one way of dealing with that fear is to pretend that everything is normal and okay. No wonder I was annoyed with the young doctor who was practicing medicine the way it ought to be practiced.

Coping with oxygen

This is not the end of the story. Denial takes some time to fade away. At least for me it did. I went through a similar process when it came to taking medication and initiating doctor's appointments. I have seen, in my own practice, how irrational thinking can cloud the judgment of people who usually function on a reasonably rational level in their everyday life. One has to overcome the irrational idea that if you have to take medicine it means you are sick, and accept the fact that you have a disease and there are medicines available to help manage it and improve your quality of life.

This is especially the case with the use of supplemental oxygen. It is difficult to overcome the idea that the less oxygen you use the less sick you are. What was helpful to me was meeting other people with pulmonary disease who were most willing to share their experiences with the use of supplemental oxygen.

I soon learned that almost everyone I met carried their own small pulse oximeter. They would monitor their oxygen saturation and came to know how many liters they needed when they were at rest, walking, or engaged in exercise. Most had encountered providers that didn't approve of their monitoring their oxygen saturation, but soon found what was helpful to them didn't always coincide with what the professional thought would be helpful.

I monitor my oxygen use, which is currently 2 liters at rest, 6 liters walking at my usual pace, and 6 to 9 liters when I work out on the bike. All are continuous flow. I had a TTO in November 2009 and feel much stronger and also have may voice back.

Me, a "patient"?

You may have noticed I have avoided use of the word, "patient." I must say that I haven't noticed any of my fellow COPDers get their dander up when someone refers to them as a patient. Part of my problem has to do with being a provider of care who is now on the receiving end. But I also think it has to do with the uneven playing field between the health professional and the patient, and the loss of autonomy that being labeled may imply.

I had not paid much attention to this until I found myself identified as the "patient" and being related to, by some, as if who you are plays second fiddle to what you got. Perhaps all health care providers ought to have a go at being a patient.

When I sit in a waiting room and hear an 80-year-old being beckoned by a youngster who looks like he just got out of high school, and who calls the patient by his first name without asking and talks to him in a tone as if he was talking to a young child, I think how infantilizing and un-empowering this is. On the surface it may seem to create a more friendly and intimate atmosphere, but on a deeper level it reinforces the loss of independent functioning as a competent adult.

This is not a trivial matter. With illness comes the inevitable loss of function. People with a chronic progressive disease, such as COPD, must learn to cope with profound loss of function to be able to deal with the feelings of depression, which can become crippling.

Sharing experiences

While there is no way to predict how any particular individual will react to being told he has a chronic disease, I can share some of my own reactions and observations. Whenever I think I've gotten past the initial denial of my illness, I am quickly reminded that denial dies hard, especially when I think I can manage some task or activity without planning ahead as to my oxygen requirements. It always is a hard reminder, and it is always a relief to know that I can manage most things with an adequate supply of oxygen.

I found the feeling of helplessness can be the cloud that overshadows every aspect of my life, or it can be the propellant to action. It can be the force that pushes one to learn as much as one can about the disease and to find out what you can do to slow it down and maintain an enjoyable quality of life, while minimizing the downtimes.

There is a wealth of information available on COPD on the Internet. However, the most helpful source of information and support for me came from other people who have COPD and who have found unique ways of living a quality and productive life. In a very real sense they empowered me to move on and to join the growing group of advocates for the study and treatment of COPD. What I was finding out firsthand was how willing people are to share their experiences and knowledge.

In talking and being with other people who have a pulmonary disease, I found that I am not the sole proprietor of denial. There's a lot of that going around. Most people get through their denial with support from family and fellow COPDers. It also seems there is consensus that the major self treatment for bouts of depression is to find ways to empower yourself, to beat the demons of helplessness and loss. None of this would be possible without the availability of a supply of portable oxygen and the groundbreaking work of Dr. Tom Petty, who dispelled some of the myths of oxygen therapy.

Overcoming stigmas

So now we come to the enormous help support groups, health care professionals, and family can provide in overcoming the stigmas, both imagined and real, in using portable oxygen in everyday living. To some the use of oxygen is a sign of weakness, proclaiming to all that there is something wrong with you and that you brought this on yourself by contaminating your lungs with smoke.

What it boiled down to for me was, there is no more denying that I am mortal and have a chronic disease. The first time I ventured out to shop for groceries while wearing my oxygen, I was self conscious, but it didn't take long to realize people were more interested in picking out the ripe melon than looking at me. In fact, I met some interesting people on the grocery line who were also on supplemental oxygen, and discovered the good feeling that comes with the sharing of information and experiences.

I have the good fortune of being able to be part of a group that is working to inform the public and health professionals about COPD. This is a group made up of health care providers, representatives from the health care industry, and yes, patients like me. As part of this group, I have met some extraordinary people who are using supplemental oxygen and are making an enormous contribution to understanding and living with COPD. Most of us were influenced by the work of Dr. Petty, who was the pioneer in the use of portable supplemental oxygen, and know how much he advocated for the sensible and adequate use of oxygen to enable people with pulmonary disease to live a quality life. In being part of this group I was able to meet and know both Dr. Petty and his collaborator, Louise Nett, who together built the foundation upon which the use of portable oxygen evolved.

Empowering leap

I hope my personal account of the psychological impact of having COPD will be helpful to those of you who are at the beginning of this process, and helpful to the health care professional who will work with you to manage this disease. As I look back on my personal odyssey, the hardest part of the journey has been hurdling the massive denial of my illness. Making this leap allowed me to empower myself and regain some sense that I could be helpful to others. The feelings of helplessness and depression faded as I joined my fellow "patients" to help other "patients" to empower themselves.

"Fish come and go, but it is the memory of afternoons on the stream that endure."
E. Donnall Thomas

Chapter 6

Oxygen Use on Vancouver Island

Christopher S. Wigley, BSc, P.Eng (Retired)

My father was a successful doctor who worked in public health. At about the time that most teenagers decide to rebel, my father became aware of the emerging statistics related to smoking and lung cancer and he decided to quit smoking, so of course I took up smoking!

I relate to things mechanical so I decided to become a mechanical engineer. As an engineer I found myself working in a variety of industrial environments – a machine shop where the oil fumes hung like a blue haze, cast iron foundry, aluminum smelter, sawmill, and steel mill. It was in the steel mill that I ended up handling the chlorine cylinders in the mill sewage plant (and got the odd whiff of chlorine) and designing an oxygen lance to feed 100 psi oxygen through a 1 1/2" pipe into a furnace at 2500 degrees!

In 1993 this steel company transferred me from Regina in Canada to the banks of the Mississippi in Iowa. Shortly after I arrived in Iowa I was diagnosed with the early stages of emphysema, which I blamed on a case of pneumonia the year before and promptly ignored the new diagnosis. My wife and I came to love Iowa, but every summer I seemed to get a terrible cough that would not clear up however many antibiotics I took.

One summer I must have been on three or four different antibiotics and was back in my doctor's office coughing again. The doctor looked thoughtful, and somewhat doubtfully offered me a sample of Singulair to "try." I took one that night and next morning the cough was gone and has never came back in the same way again. Singulair is really supposed to be an asthma drug but, although I have always suffered from hayfever and have several people in my family with asthma, I had never had an asthma attack or even wheezed much.

My job involved both a lot of desk work as well as quality supervision in all areas of the plant. As time went on I found the "in-plant" work more and more difficult - poor air quality in the plant plus catwalks and stairways to get over and being around all the conveying equipment - so I delegated more and more of this work to my "second-in-command" and spent even more of my days doing the desk work. Little did I realize at the time that this was the classic downward spiral of breathlessness causing lack of exercise and resulting in less fitness and so more breathlessness and so less exercise. My boss wanted me out in the plant more and decided to fire me – call it early retirement!

My wife was still working in a good job, so I became "Mr Mom" for a while doing most of the shopping, cleaning and cooking. I started doing more research on my "emphysema" and discovered it was really COPD and not just early stage of emphysema. I was getting really short of breath when I was doing anything active, such as cutting the grass in the ditch in front of the house. I had even talked to my doctor about getting oxygen, but he just prescribed another albuterol (known in Canada as salbutamol) inhaler.

I started looking into where we should retire. For us it was a "no-brainer" to return to Canada both for the health system and because we had no family in the US, but a daughter in Winnipeg and a son in Victoria, on Vancouver Island. I made a couple of trips to scout out the possibilities – neither my wife nor I are fond of big cities so I looked around outside of Winnipeg, but the thought of the winters on the prairie with the snow and wind was more than I felt a couple of 'old-timers' would want to handle. So I turned my attention to Vancouver Island. It is truly one of the most beautiful places on earth, with basically a very mild climate – not too hot in summer or too cold in winter. It seemed perfect — never too far from the sea but with beautiful tree-covered mountains, mostly capped in snow during the winter. I started looking for a house suitable for a retired couple - think single level, preferably handicap accessible, etc. I ended up buying almost the opposite - two levels and with a ridiculously steep driveway with the house a good 20 feet above road level, but a beautiful location. I arranged to rent it out until we could move back to Canada when my wife retired.

During this period of being "Mr Mom" I actually did fairly well at the cooking even going as far as making an almost perfect Tiramisu[1] dessert. I suspect that this was my downfall as very shortly after this I began getting really short of breath and had some spells feeling really sick with a lot of sweating. My doctor sent me for a stress test and the cardiologist supervising the test stopped it before the first minute was up and told me to report at the hospital the next day for an angiogram. Apparently I had had a couple of silent heart attacks, resulting in two of the three arteries feeding the heart being totally blocked! Luckily I had some parallel circulation from the third artery preventing any permanent damage. However, since this episode my wife has banned me from ever eating Tiramisu again!

After I had a couple of stents put in I was enrolled in a cardiac rehab program and started, for the first time in my life, to look at exercise as something almost enjoyable! However I did think to get the cardio therapists to check my oxygen saturation levels when I was exercising. The result was that I was told not to exercise so hard as my saturation was dropping below 90% - when I asked why I couldn't get oxygen (some of the other heart patients were on oxygen) I was firmly told that I didn't want that as it would make me retain CO_2 and then I would stop breathing! There are still so many medical professionals who believe this myth! I did however manage to get my doctor to arrange for a pulmonary function test. The pulmonologist who read the results found a post-bronchodilator FEV_1 of just over 30% and diagnosed severe COPD. By this time I was almost finished with my cardio rehab and I was able to switch directly over from cardio to pulmonary rehab.

My Adventure with Oxygen

As usual with pulmonary rehab, the first thing was the six minute walk test for the RT to evaluate my current condition, and then on to a treadmill. I think it was no more than a minute on the treadmill before the RT handed me a cannula and started me on my new adventure with oxygen. I took some time to decide what oxygen equipment would be most suitable for me and my lifestyle. I even toyed with the idea of using welding oxygen from a welding supply place, but soon ruled that out as I would still need suitable regulators and cannulas, etc. I looked very closely at the Chad Total O2 setup with a concentrator/compressor/tank filling combination but ended up choosing a Helios liquid portable system with a concentrator to use at night. The concentrator, reservoir and Helios were delivered by Apria on Christmas Eve 2003. Some Christmas present, although my wife tells me that at the time I was not too happy about having to use oxygen!

This worked very well for me, allowing me total mobility during the daytime. With the Helios in a waist-pack I had both hands free to carry shopping bags and open doors at the same time. I could get into the car and just drive off without having to put a tank in a safe place within reach of the cannula while getting a cannula caught up on everything that stuck out!

I soon started to find some of the drawbacks to this set-up for me. The first was that, as a result of an operation to one of my ears, I could not get a cannula to stay in place – there was not enough ear at the top to hold a cannula securely in place! I solved that, at least during the daytime, by getting Oxy-View glasses. These wonderful eyeglass frames have a tiny metal tube in place of the normal side arms of the glasses to feed the oxygen through. But these did not do well with the Helios portable oxygen, so I ended up changing the Helios for a Spirit 300 which uses a single lumen 'cannula' in place of the dual lumen of the Helios. An added advantage of this is that the Spirit is less prone to freezing than the Helios and also gives a better and larger bolus (puff) of oxygen at each breath. The second was to use soft-hose cannulas (www.softhose.com) at night – these lovely soft cannulas mold to the contours of the face and seem to want to cling to the skin. They simply stay on better. Also you can custom order to whatever length you like. When I use these with my Spirit I use a really short cannula that hangs close to my body – in five years I do not think I have caught one on a door-knob or drawer handle more than half-a-dozen times! Nor have I ever tripped over an oxygen hose – and more of my on-line friends than I care to think about have tripped over an oxygen hose, fallen, and broken bones.

The cost of the oxygen in the US has always frustrated me – I know that a large part of the cost of home oxygen is supposed to be for home care and supplies – but I was buying my own supplies, and the only time I saw an RT from the supplier was when one was instructed, by my health insurance, to come and check how fast I breathed! I checked on E-Bay and bought a couple of low hours concentrators for a couple of hundred dollars each – five years later they are still running. If I remember correctly this saved me about $40 a month co-pay – not a bad investment. I was also thinking that I would be retiring to Vancouver Island in a year or two and I had heard that it was hard to get approved for oxygen in Canada.

Another of the things that I learned early on was that a steady flow of dry O2 in the nose can be very uncomfortable. Putting a humidifier on the concentrator eased this tremendously, but then I ended up with condensation in the tubing – especially in winter and I kept the concentrator downstairs but slept upstairs so I had a long hose! Obviously the solution was to put the humidifier beside the bed instead of on the concentrator, so I made a wooden frame to hold a humidifier, with a hospital type flowmeter on top, a mini heater underneath from an old coffee mug warmer and, just to top it off and because the bedside table was small, I mounted my alarm clock on top as well. You can see a picture at http://s212.photobucket.com/albums/cc58/wigleyc/ The heater turned out to be a huge overkill!

That year I took a vacation in England. I arranged for oxygen on the flight, but rented (then a brand-new invention) – a Portable Oxygen Concentrator to use while in England. This was an AirSep Lifestyle which worked well for me, even at night, but had a pitifully short operating time on the battery – I spent a lot of time looking for places to plug in and charge up! It was interesting to see the reaction of the doctors in our family, as they were not accustomed to seeing active people on oxygen, let alone a portable concentrator! As soon as the Inogen came out, I broke open the piggy bank and bought an Inogen which had about 3 hours or more battery life. Inogen has been wonderful about updating and warranty repair (once) and I still use this when flying, or travelling.

As it got closer to my wife's retiring we started to think about our move to Vancouver Island. We would be moving into a much smaller house, and most of our furniture would not suit or fit, but there were a lot of personal things such as books, photographs, and personal things that we did not want to leave behind. We also wanted to move as cheaply as possible, so I decided to buy a used small moving van, and do all the packing and loading myself.

As part of the planning for the big move I checked for oxygen on Vancouver Island. I could find only two companies that handled liquid oxygen on the island, and neither had anything like the Spirit or even a Helios – the only portable liquid oxygen equipment appeared to be 'Strollers.' Now I have nothing against 'Strollers,' but they would not give me the freedom and mobility that a Spirit does, so I talked to Apria and arranged to buy the

Spirit from them, and return the liquid reservoir to their Seattle office when we drove through on the way to the Vancouver Island ferry. I also arranged with a local oxygen company on Vancouver Island for another full reservoir to be waiting for us at my son's house in Victoria. They were happy to do this with a prescription from my doctor in Iowa. Of course after a few weeks we got a bill for $833!

As soon as we arrived on Vancouver Island, I checked in with the doctor to arrange prescriptions for all the usual COPD (and heart) drugs and, of course, the oxygen. This also involves arranging for provincial health coverage (in Canada the Federal Government-mandated universal health care coverage, but the coverage is provided by each province, with each province having different regulations). The medical plan (covering doctor and hospital costs) is about $300 quarterly for two people. Drug coverage has a deductible (which varies depending on the income tax paid in the previous year) and different "tier" costs for preferred drugs.

Home oxygen is covered in a different way. It is covered in full for everyone who qualifies, but supplemental health insurance (for non-essential medical care such as private rooms in hospitals, full drug coverage, etc.) you are required to pay your share where people have this insurance. The problem comes with the qualification conditions for home oxygen. The conditions are very specific and change somewhat from time to time, but at that time an arterial blood gas (ABG) had to be less than 55 mm Hg on room air, or between 56 and 59 with evidence of congestive heart failure or polycythemia. Oxygen for exertion had to demonstrate desaturation below 85% saturation of oxygen (SaO2) with slow recovery and who have underlying disease or below 80% regardless of distance walked or dyspnea. Oxygen for sleep was an ABG during the day between 55 and 60 and SaO2 less than 90% for more than 15% of the night.

I went for the arterial blood gas analysis on the 2nd floor of the local hospital and walked up the stairs without my portable O2 and presented at the RT's office flourishing my oximeter showing 78% thinking "this should short-cut a whole bunch of other testing." NOT. The RT's only job was to get the ABG. So after 20 minutes on room air he did the blood draw and found 81 mmHg, which didn't qualify. The next day I showed up at the O2 supplier for them to do the exertion test. We walked around for ten minutes without oxygen and after 4 minutes I was down to an SaO2 of about 81%

and even dropped to 79% for half a minute. AHA! I qualified on two grounds! So the paperwork was sent off to the Home Oxygen Program (HOP) office and a week later I was told that I did not qualify. I did some researching and found out the name of someone at the HOP office and called, explaining the test results and the decline for funding. The gentleman promised to look into it and get back to me. A week later he did and apologized that they had made a mistake and I did indeed qualify!

Three months later I got a home visit for the HOP three month review by the HOP's own RT and got another ABG and walk test. This time there was a blind test walking with O2 and with compressed air to see whether the oxygen actually helped. Again I passed the tests, but got another letter saying I didn't qualify — another series of phone calls and another apology for a "mistake." It appears the respirologist (Canadian speak for pulmonologist!) who had to approve the subsidy had a tendency to make 'mistakes.' Some people wondered whether his salary bonus was related to the number of people he was able to deny subsidy to!

As we settled into our new home, periodically visiting my son who lived in Victoria for the weekend, we found it actually more convenient to pick up our liquid oxygen in our mini-van, using a 21 litre tank (which typically lasts me about 12 days), than have them deliver the big tank which was too big and heavy for me to man-handle into the van. This seems to work out well for us, as well as being more convenient for the oxygen supplier, who didn't have any other deliveries in our area.

Things settled in pretty well after that. I still love my Caire Spirit. I really wanted another as a back-up and found one at a good price on E-bay. It was a good thing I did, because I got caught in a good rainstorm when out with my Spirit. The rain got into the 'works' and it stopped pulsing. My local O2 supplier doesn't handle the Spirit, so it was time to put into effect my mechanical engineers' motto "if you can't open it up, then you don't own it." Apart it came and I learned just how it works and what needed fixing. The folks in the Caire service department are wonderful and shipped me the parts needed to fix it, and it now works better than ever!

I started a local COPD support group as there was neither a local pulmonary rehab nor any other support group in Duncan. I wish I could say that it is a howling success, but there is a steady core of half a dozen or so regulars (when they are not being 'snowbirds' and flocking off to Arizona to chase the sun) and a thin but steady stream of new members. We have no respirologist in town, and most of the local GPs seem oblivious to fact that the disease is TREATABLE and far less that a support group or rehab might help.

In 2006 I heard about the Canadian COPD Alliance conference in Calgary and decided to register myself and go to the conference. I found that there was indeed a large body of the medical profession that was very up-to-date and upbeat about treating COPD. I was the one and only patient among what seemed like 1000 respirologists and RTs but I left inspired at their universal acknowledgement of the importance of exercise in COPD. However, I was also puzzled that there seemed to be no realization that COPDers, with low oxygen levels with exercise, are simply not going to exercise the way that they are capable of without good portable oxygen available. While there I met with Nora Sobolov, the president of the Canadian Lung Association, who told me about the Canadian Lung Health Framework and told me that she would like me to become involved.

Sometime in the following few months I met Jackie Whitaker of Nova Scotia on the internet and joined the fledgling Canadian internet support group for people with COPD (COPD Canada Patient Network – (www.copdcanada.ca) and ended up as the vice-president of this organization. Jackie had started this as a web site only for World COPD Day in 2006 and then developed it into the thriving internet support group that it is today.

As a member of the board of COPD Canada Patient Network, I have been a delegate on the interim steering committee of the Canadian 'Lung Health Framework.' That in itself is another story entirely, but it has meant that I have needed to travel several times from Victoria to Ottawa, and once to Vancouver.

As a patient with severe COPD and on oxygen this means that I definitely need oxygen when flying. As you go higher the air becomes thinner and each breath you take in contains less molecules of oxygen. The pressure in a modern jet plane is the equivalent of an elevation of 8,000 ft (2,500 metres), so even some people who do not need oxygen at sea level, may need it when flying.

Living with oxygen always takes some planning, but a trip by plane and a stay for a week or so in another city takes a lot more than a visit to the corner store! Living in Canada is not always the easiest for those on oxygen, but where flying is concerned, it is truly much easier. This is because West-Jet operates here, and they not only treat their passengers extremely well but they also fully recognize and allow for the needs of passengers on oxygen. They simply allow users to bring on board their own oxygen systems (only on flights that do not leave Canada) or portable oxygen concentrators!

You are allowed up to two systems, which could be two tank systems (regulators may not be changed while on board the plane) or portable oxygen concentrator, but not liquid systems such as a Helios. Planning also involves arranging for oxygen at your destination (I used Medigas in Ottawa, a prescription for the oxygen was needed but they obtained a copy from my local supplier), and a prescription from my doctor on a special form from Westjet. Other airlines are likely to have a similar requirement.

I normally use a Caire Spirit liquid oxygen system, but this is not allowed for in flight use. So for my first trip I arranged to stay the night before at my son's house and then for him to drive me to the airport. The plan was to use the Spirit until I got to the airport to save on the Inogen batteries, then switch to the Inogen and keep my one cylinder (in a hydration backpack) as a backup in case the two batteries would not last the full time.

On arrival at the airport I planned to pack my Spirit in my checked baggage and switch to my Inogen for most of the rest of the journey. Those of you who use liquid oxygen can probably imagine this next scene. To pack the Spirit in my baggage would mean that I would have to vent out the liquid oxygen from the Spirit. So there I am, standing outside the main door to the terminal, and I take my spirit and open the vent valve - clouds of white gas now surrounds me and the other passengers at the Departure entrance to the terminal. And the security personnel and RCMP start moving in!!!!

I am very lucky that my son, a civilian member of the RCMP, knew the RCMP officer and was able to explain that I was just venting some harmless oxygen. Otherwise I might still be incarcerated awaiting trial for terrorist acts! I really don't blame the check-in people, but they would not let me put the now empty spirit in my checked baggage! I think I was lucky even to get on that plane!

After that experience I just used the Inogen to get to the airport. I checked with Transport Canada (Canadian equivalent of the FAA) and with the head of the safety for Westjet and I now have a letter saying that it is safe to pack an empty liquid oxygen portable in checked baggage provided that the vent valve is kept open.

A total of about five hours flying time with at least one stopover is really pushing it with only two batteries for the Inogen, and I would not have attempted it without the cylinder back-up. At the stops rushing to find an outlet to recharge the batteries between flights, and as you can't leave baggage unattended that meant only a quick visit to the washroom and no coffee (though I did once persuade the gate personnel to watch my bag for a couple of minutes). At times like this I find being on oxygen very limiting.

I was able to just slide the Inogen with it's wheeled cart and minipack for charger and spare battery, as well as the hydration pack with the M-6 cylinder under the seat in front of me. This still left room for my feet but hardly any room to even wiggle my toes!

In flight I used my oximeter to watch my sats and tried to maintain an SaO2 about 90%. This was fine although it needed occasional pursed lip breathing until I cranked up the flow rate as we ascended. However bending over in that confined space (and I admit to being a little overweight) to change batteries was pretty unpleasant. First the concentrator shuts down, then you need to remove the battery, get out the spare battery, put away the old battery, put the new battery in and then restart the concentrator all while bent double and with no oxygen just at a time when you really need at least a couple more liters/min than usual. Kinda makes bending over to tie up a pair of shoelaces seem like a walk in the park (actually even walks in the park aren't as easy as they used to be!).

The other thing that really caught me by surprise, and I think is something that has not been properly considered, is that there is less of a sensation of being short of breath than usual. I suspect that this is related to that lower pressure at altitude tending to help the body get rid of excess $CO2$ from the blood, and it is of course the raised blood $CO2$ levels above our own normal levels that drive us to feel breathless. It was really brought home to me when I glanced at my little Nonin oximeter after waking from a short nap and saw my O2 level had dropped to 80%. I do not have sleep apnea and did not have a problem maintaining 90% when awake and keeping an eye on that little Nonin. I really recommend a finger oximeter when flying.

My other flight was to Vancouver by float plane. I love flying in small planes as you see so much more and there is more sensation of actually flying. This was on a small single engine Beaver (50 years old to the day when I made the flight!) owned by a local air taxi firm. I wondered whether they would mind about flying with O2, but they knew what portable oxygen concentrators were and had no problem with my using my Inogen.

Although travelling with oxygen can sometimes be challenging, with good planning it is definitely doable and that can allow one's life to be much more satisfying. Did I mention that two of my granddaughters live in Ottawa? My wife and I have also done a cruise to Alaska with SeaPuffers, and are planning another to the Caribbean, flying to Florida for the cruise, and then returning to Vancouver Island (with a couple of stops to visit internet friends) all the way via Amtrak. It should be quite an adventure.

For the record my FEV_1 when first tested was 28% pre and 33% post bronchodilator, and I do not think it has changed much since it was first tested in 2002, but I have not had it checked since. I was first prescribed O2 at 2 l/min at rest and sleeping and 4 l/min with exercise, and have not had a respirologist change the prescription since (but I "Titrate as I Migrate"[2]). Just sitting without O2 (and at 500' elevation) I am typically 90 -92% SaO2. I try to maintain my sats around 92% minimum. I do not normally have a wet cough and do not tend to notice if my O2 sats drop significantly. My usual first symptoms of low SaO2 are slight feeling of inebriation (woozy and unsteady) and very painful calf muscles if this is when walking.

---

1. Tiramesù " [tirame su]) is one of the most popular Italian cakes. It is made of savoiardi (otherwise known as lady finger biscuits) dipped in espresso or strong coffee or rum, layered with a whipped mixture of egg yolks, mascarpone, and sugar, and topped with cocoa.

2. Available for free download at: http://www.perf2ndwind.org/html/tompetty/2006/Nov-2006.html

Chapter 7

Transtracheal Oxygen Therapy:

The Best Kept Secret in Pulmonary Medicine?

John R. Goodman, B.S., RRT

Transtracheal oxygen therapy (TTOT) is the administration of oxygen directly into the trachea (windpipe) via a small, flexible, plastic catheter. It is intended only for patients requiring long term, continuous oxygen therapy. It has proven to be a scientifically valid alternative to oxygen delivered by a standard nasal cannula.

LTOT has been utilized to treat a variety of pulmonary conditions since the 1930's. Early work by Richards and Barach,[1,2] and later Petty and Finigan,[3] suggested that oxygen therapy could significantly benefit selected COPD patients. Current estimates suggest that there are somewhere between 800,000 and 1.2 million patients receiving continuous supplemental oxygen. The cost of this therapy exceeds 2-3 billion dollars per year.[4] The vast majority of these patients use a nasal cannula for their oxygen delivery. Nasal cannulae are inexpensive and simple to use, but compliance with nasal oxygen is suboptimal for a variety of reasons.

Landmark studies such as the Nocturnal Oxygen Therapy Trial (NOTT) done in the 1970's clearly showed that nasal cannula patients were actually willing or able to wear their oxygen less than 18 hours per day.[5] When these patients were asked about their non-compliance, the complained of discomfort wearing the nasal cannula, and occasional dislodgment of the cannula during sleep. Additionally, many patients will not go out in public wearing a nasal cannula because of self-consciousness or embarrassment. The net result of this non-compliance is that many (if not most) oxygen dependent patients are *not* getting the full benefit of their oxygen therapy, and the majority of patients are not able to follow their oxygen prescription as intended by their physician.

In an attempt to eliminate the problems inherent in the design of the nasal cannula, Henry Heimlich M.D. created the concept of delivering oxygen directly into the trachea. Dr. Heimlich published his findings on 100 patients in 1982. In his study, Dr. Heimlich reported few complications, a reduction of about 50% in the patients resting oxygen flow rate, and most patients reported improvements in both their shortness of breath and ability to ambulate.[6]

In 1984 two Denver area physicians (Bryan Spofford, ENT surgeon and Kent Christopher MD RRT) combined their different areas of expertise and developed what became known as the SCOOP transtracheal oxygen program of care.[7] The chief reason the "SCOOP" catheter has survived 20+ years, while a number of other catheters have come and gone, is the fact that TTO using the SCOOP catheter had been conceived as a "program" of care from the very beginning. The actual procedure, while important, is just one part of the larger overall program of care.

Benefits of Transtracheal Oxygen Therapy

With nearly a quarter of a century of experience in patients from all around the world, the benefits of TTOT are very well known. In fact, TTOT offers many of the benefits, which meet the specific therapeutic goals of the NOTT study. True 24-hour compliance with oxygen therapy, a more active lifestyle, and conservation of oxygen resources are all feasible with TTOT. The average TTOT patient has a 50-60% reduction in resting oxygen flow rate, and a 30% decrease with activity.[7] TTOT can be used very effectively with pulse or dose type oxygen conserving devices. It is very important to note however, that if a TTOT patient is going to use an oxygen-conserving device, it MUST be of a single lumen design. Obviously with a transtracheal catheter, there is only one way in and one way out. Therefore a device such as the Helios liquid oxygen canister will NOT work with a transtracheal catheter. A very good alternative would be the Spirit 300 as it is a single lumen design and almost identical to the Helios in size and weight.

The combined physiologic and mechanical benefits of transtracheal oxygen result in an improved overall quality of life for the patient. Additionally, in at least one study, transtracheal patients lived longer than matched nasal cannula patients.[11] In fact, they lived over 24 months longer than their nasal cannula counterparts. Even to the layperson this seems logical since TTOT patients actually do get their oxygen every minute of every hour of every day. Remember, if you are better oxygenated ALL major organ systems of the body are better oxygenated. This includes your heart, brain, liver, kidneys, pancreas etc. Other studies of TTOT have documented reduced hospitalizations, reduced shortness of breath, and as already mentioned increased longevity.[8,9,10,11] It's easy to overlook how much discomfort is associated with wearing a nasal cannula, yet this is the number one reason patients list for being non-compliant. Similarly, it is easy to underestimate how embarrassing wearing a nasal cannula in public is for some patients. Once a patient is receiving transtracheal oxygen, both of these problems are quickly eliminated, thereby adding immeasurably to the patient's quality of life.

The SCOOP Program of Care

The word SCOOP is actually an acronym for Spofford …Christopher…Oxygen …Optimizing…Program. SCOOP is **not** just a procedure, but a program of care that requires a systematic team approach to produce the best results for the patient. A knowledgeable team consists of a physician, surgeon, office or hospital based respiratory therapist (RT) or nurse, the patient and their partner, and the patient's home care company. Together they provide the education, clinical support and supplies necessary to support transtracheal patients during the four phases of the program. In this way, all of the special needs of the pulmonary patient, in addition to their oxygen requirements will be periodically monitored for appropriateness. The SCOOP program basically divides itself into four clinical phases, which will be described briefly below.

Phase 1: Patient Orientation, Evaluation, Selection, and Preparation.

There are a number of goals associated with each phase of the SCOOP program. In Phase 1 the goals include:

Patient education.
Identification of indications and precautions.

Identification of good candidates and exclusion of poor candidates. Stabilization of the patient before the procedure.

Phase 1 is unquestionably the most important of the four clinical phases. In phase 1 potential transtracheal patients are oriented, evaluated, selected, and prepared for the transtracheal procedure. Patients may hear about TTOT from a variety of sources. This may include the patient's physician, family member or friend, another transtracheal patient, or through various types of advertising. If the patient is enrolled in a pulmonary rehabilitation program, they may well have heard about TTOT from the respiratory therapist who leads the group sessions. As patients become more and more Internet savvy, there are many portals available for patient seeking information on TTOT. A number of very active Internet patient support groups are available as well.

A case for "realistic expectations."

While it is true that TTOT can provide better and more efficient oxygenation than a nasal cannula, TTOT is NOT a lung transplant. The lung disease you have before a SCOOP procedure is exactly the same after the procedure. Keeping your expectations realistic is very, very important. This goes for the whole health care team as well. Perhaps an example might be helpful here. Suppose we have a patient in San Diego getting 4 L/min using a nasal cannula. While sitting quietly in his/her favorite easy chair, his finger pulse oximeter shows his oxygen saturation to bounce back and forth between 90 and 91%. While many clinicians and patients might say this patient is doing all right, in reality, his oxygen saturation should be somewhere in the mid to high 90's at least. This patient should really be on a higher resting flow rate sufficient to keep his oxygen saturations at 95% or better. If this patient thinks his/her flow rate will drop 50% to around 2 L/min, because of what he has read or been told, he/she will be upset when this is not the case. In this example, the patient's *transtracheal flow rate* might be 3 or even 4 L/min…but the patient will be very well saturated. The goal of TTOT in all patients is to adequately oxygenate the patient first, and secondarily to conserve or use less oxygen. It is extremely important that patients, their families and their TTOT team remain aware of this fact so that preconceived expectations have a much better chance of being met.

With tens of thousands of months of experience over the years, which types of patients do best with TTOT have been very well identified. Experience gained from patients all around the world has proven that the following patients do best with TTOT.

Patients who are currently using between 1-6 L/min via nasal cannula with acceptable oxygen saturations. i.e. Resting O2 saturations in the mid-90's.

Patients who have reasonable pulmonary function values.

Patients who have stable arterial blood gases.

Patients who have dependable transportation and do not live very far from the hospital, doctor, respiratory therapist or nurse who is doing the post procedure education and follow-up.

Patients who have a strong, competent, and committed partner or other family support.

Patients who spend less than 12 hours per day in bed.

Patients who leave the house routinely for activities such as shopping, socializing, working etc

Patients who are highly motivated to improve the quality of their life. These are patients who just know there must be a better way to get their oxygen.

Among the most difficult patients seeking transtracheal oxygen are those with very high oxygen flow rates, or end stage disease. This may create an emotional situation for the referring physician who may have been taking care of this patient for many years. There is a great deal of pressure to "do something." Honest evaluation and frank discussion between the physician, the patient and their family can help with some of these very difficult situations. TTOT achieves the best results when used *early* in the progression of the disease. Roughly 80% of all current TTOT patients have COPD as their primary underlying disease. Interstitial lung disease (ILD), pulmonary fibrosis, (IPF) pulmonary hypertension (PH), and other even more rare pulmonary diseases, make up the other 20% of TTOT patients.

A special note should be made here regarding the ever expanding group of diseases that fall under the umbrella of Pulmonary Fibrosis, also known a Interstitial lung disease (ILD). Although there are many identified causes of ILD, the net result is virtually the same. Patients with ILD have extreme difficulty getting oxygen to cross the barrier between their tiny air sacs, and the blood supply just beyond. ILD is progressive, and many times results in the need for very high flows of nasal oxygen. Patients with ILD "work" very hard just to breathe. TTOT can help these patients by reducing the work of breathing, while doing a better job of oxygenation than could possibly by accomplished by the nasal cannula. A word of warning regarding realistic expectations: Due to the nature of the disease, reducing the resting oxygen flow rate by approximately 50% *is* commonly seen. However, with even limited physical activity, the patient's oxygen saturation will probably still fall to very low levels. On the positive side, recovery back to baseline levels is generally much faster. Additionally, the ILD patient (like all TTOT patients) will be much more comfortable without the nasal cannula at high flows, (probably unhumidified) on their face. It is especially important for both the patient and TTO team to have clinically realistic expectations when evaluating an ILD patient for TTOT.

Phase 2: The Transtracheal procedure itself

The goals of Phase 2 are quite simple and include:

> The creation of a quality tract (opening) into the trachea and,
> Making sure the patient is medically stable on the day of the procedure, monitored throughout the night following the procedure, and during the week that follows.

Currently there are two very different techniques for initiating transtracheal oxygen. The older technique involves a simple outpatient procedure. As an outpatient procedure it is normally done using only local anesthetic. It takes about 30 minutes to perform and the patient goes home the same day. Although the opening is very small, it takes approximately 6-8 weeks to heal completely. During this time patients are routinely seen once a week to monitor the progress of the healing, and to educate the patient regarding the daily cleaning of the catheter. The catheter *must* remain in the tract during this entire period of time. Once the tract is fully healed, the patient is taught how to remove one catheter and insert a clean catheter once or twice a day. This procedure is based on a time proven technique known as the "Modified Seldinger" technique or MST.

Alternatively, a procedure called "Fast Tract" was developed to shorten the healing time required by the MST. It is a surgical procedure that is performed in the operating room by a qualified surgeon. The Fast Tract procedure is done by an Otolaryngologist about 99% of the time, although a Cardiothoracic or General surgeon is certainly qualified to do the Fast Tract procedure. Since IV medication will be used for patient comfort, an anesthesiologist must be in attendance. The procedure takes about 45 minutes to an hour and the patient spends the night in the hospital. There are a number of advantages to the Fast Tract procedure. Transtracheal oxygen is initiated the very next day instead of one week later as in the MST. Also, the normal 6-8 week period of time necessary for a fully healed tract is reduced to 10-14 days, significantly reducing minor complications.

The decision regarding which of the two procedures is best for the patient depends on a number of variables, and varies from patient to patient. The patient and physician should make the final decision with input from the family if necessary. Due to its significant advantages over the older MST, the Fast Tract procedure has unquestionably become the procedure of choice among surgeons doing transtracheal procedures throughout the United States.

Phase 3: Waiting for the transtracheal tract to heal

As before there are several goals that must be accomplished in Phase 3. They include:

The initiation of transtracheal oxygen therapy.

Avoiding and/or treating any problems with mucus management or tract problems.

Educating and supporting the patient during this phase.

Whether the procedure was done using the MST or Fast Tract approach, transtracheal oxygen is actually started in Phase 3. The "stent" or placeholder that was inserted during the procedure can now be removed over a wire guide, and a functioning SCOOP catheter can be placed into the tract. Phase 3 normally lasts 6-8 weeks with the MST and about 2 weeks with the Fast Tract procedure. During this time the patient cleans the catheter in place with saline irrigation and the use of a specifically designed cleaning rod. This is normally done twice a day, but may be increased by a transtracheal team member based on clinical observation. Normally, the patient is taught how to clean and care for their catheter by a respiratory therapist or nurse. Every new TTOT patient receives a full set of written instructional materials, as well as several DVDs that show the patient exactly what is expected of them regarding their cleaning protocols.

Patients are educated regarding the possible development of mucus problems, how to recognize them, and what to do if suspected. Mucus problems are largely preventable and in all cases easy to treat *if brought to the attention of designated team personnel.* An occasional tract problem may also develop during phase 3. These too are normally very easy to identify and treat. Most treatments involve antibiotic administration and review of cleaning techniques. Approximately 95% of Seldinger created tracts are fully healed by 6 weeks. An occasional patient may require one or two more weeks before complete healing is achieved. Fast Tract patients typically find their tract fully healed by the beginning of the third week from the date of their stent placement. With either procedure, patients move from Phase 3 to Phase 4 when their tract is fully healed.

Phase 3 is the most challenging of the four phases, as this is when minor complications are most likely to develop. A skilled team can anticipate most of these problems and either prevent them or treat them safely and routinely as they occur.

Phase 4: Transtracheal Oxygen with a completely healed tract.

The goals of Phase 4 include the following:

Making sure the tract is completely healed.
Designing a customized cleaning protocol.

Provide ongoing monitoring and education for the patient.

Phase 4 begins about 6-8 weeks after the MST procedure and approximately 14 days after the Fast Tract procedure. The tract should now be healed enough to permit the catheter to be removed and reinserted by the patient. This is the endpoint we are looking for. In your written materials and on the instructional DVD you may see this referred to as a fully "matured" tract.

A tract is indeed fully matured when the SCOOP catheter can be easily removed and reinserted by the patient. This is usually determined by a team member first using the wire guide, and then just the catheter alone. All patients beginning Phase 4 must show that they are capable of removing and reinserting the catheter before they are allowed to go home from this first visit of phase 4. Assessing the healing process is much less problematic with the Fast Tract technique because more tissue is removed, and the skin opening is quite a bit larger than the tract created by the MST.

The first week of Phase 4 is considered a "trial" period. If for any reason difficulty is encountered with catheter removal or reinsertion, the SCOOP catheter is reinserted and the patient continues Phase 3 for an additional 1-2 weeks. The tract can be reassessed at that time. It would be very unusual for a tract to not be fully healed following two more weeks of Phase 3 and cleaning in place again.

Medicare reimbursement for transtracheal oxygen therapy products

Reimbursement for transtracheal oxygen therapy has always been limited. There are well-established codes for the physician components; however, Medicare has determined that replacement supplies (two catheters and a SCOOP hose every 3 months) are to be included in the monthly allowable for oxygen supplies. In other words Medicare does not recognize the rather substantial difference between a simple nasal cannula and a transtracheal catheter. Oxygen reimbursement has been "modality neutral" for quite some time. This is certainly unfair to home oxygen companies and puts them in an untenable position when it comes to supplying their TTOT patients with replacement catheters and hoses. In fact, it would literally take an act of Congress to change the current lack of reimbursement, and no change in this situation is seriously being contemplated. You should tell your home oxygen company if you are considering becoming a transtracheal oxygen patient. They need to know you will require ongoing supplies, and it is better to know in advance how this is going to be handled so there are no surprises a few months down the road.

Advanced Applications of TTOT and Future Directions.

Almost from the very beginning, there have been anecdotal reports from transtracheal patients who reported that it was easier to breathe after placement of their SCOOP catheter. Patients frequently reported that they were sleeping better, had more energy during the day and had significant improvements in activities of daily living. Patients were also delighted to observe that even though they still got short of breath with increased activity, they recovered much more quickly. As the anecdotal experience grew among an increasing TTO patient population, speculation grew that indeed, if higher flow rates of an air/oxygen blend could be safely and comfortably introduced into the trachea, that further improvements in both oxygenation AND ventilation might be realized.

So far three distinct clinical applications have been studied. These advanced applications are called Transtracheal Augmented Ventilation, and is abbreviated TTAV. TTAV seems to have powerful positive effects in the following areas:

As an aid to breathing for patients with chronic respiratory insufficiency. (BiPAP users). You may remember Dr. Petty chatting with a TTAV patient in the first edition of Adventures of an Oxy-Phile (page 28).

As an aid in weaning long-term ventilator dependent patients from mechanical ventilators.

In the treatment of patients with Obstructive Sleep Apnea (OSA) who can't or won't comply with standard CPAP/BiPAP therapy.

A more thorough explanation of these three applications is beyond the scope of this chapter. Much of the success of TTAV is due to the fact that the tip of the transtracheal catheter is roughly in the same position as the tip of an endotracheal tube. Therefore, a transtracheal catheter is in excellent position to deliver not only oxygen and air alone or in combination, but also other therapeutic gases such as Heliox and Nitric Oxide. The administration of these gases transtracheally has the potential to improve the delivery of these gases directly to the lungs and enhance their effect in a wide variety of clinical conditions.

A great deal of further study needs to be performed in order to evaluate which patients are most likely to benefit from TTAV. Technical application aspects need to be refined so that commercially available TTAV delivery devices are both patient and clinician friendly, as well as economically viable. As always, questions regarding reimbursement will have to be answered in conjunction with the development of any new technology.

In the long run, TTAV may prove to be a brand new mode of augmented ventilation that physicians can consider when they have patients who are easily oxygenated at low oxygen flow rates, yet continue to complain of dyspnea and increased work of breathing. TTAV may well become the answer to the most common presenting complaint of a COPD patient on oxygen telling his pulmonologist, "But Doc, I'd be fine if I could just breathe."

Patient Testimonials:

As we have seen above, only transtracheal patients are in a position to best experience *all* the benefits long-term oxygen can bring. Proven scientifically, and published in the most respected medical journals, these benefits include living longer lives with fewer hospitalizations, and an overall better quality of life. Three patients representing 3 different clinical histories have volunteered to tell their stories.

Patient Number 1.

Sherry is a delightful 65-year-old patient who lives near Nashville, Tennessee. She has been receiving transtracheal oxygen for the past 11 years and these are her own words:

"I was diagnosed with the big "E" in 1998. Along with this news I was told my life was over and the grim prediction of no real quality of life was now mine. I would be put on oxygen and use a nose hose to breathe. Femininity was gone. Being able to breathe did work, but I felt like a freak on display.......people would stare.

"On a visit to my pulmonary doctor, she asked, "Where is your oxygen?" I replied, "It is in the car." I will never forget her words. "Well it's really helping you breathe out there isn't it?" I felt like a complete idiot. After that I never went without it again. I'm vain, but that was just stupid. That is how I got over people looking at me. I needed to breathe worse than someone rudely gawking at me.

"My pulmonary doctor suggested a "Pulmonary Rehab Program" at the Dayani Center at Vanderbilt. I took the full 6-week pulmonary rehabilitation course. It also incorporates graduated exercises that are closely monitored by respiratory therapists, and education, which is a necessary and vital component. You learn you aren't the only one with this disease and that classmates had the same feelings I did. Interaction with other patients helps a great deal. You learn how to better function in life. It was tough but well worth the effort. It dramatically improved my pulmonary function status along with the exercise. Later, after I got "SCOOPED," I re-entered Pulmonary Rehab and the pulmonary rehab staff were amazed at the improvement in my numbers between my first rehab (pre-TTOT) and my second session (post-TTOT). No more gasping for air. My workouts were so smooth, and indeed I was a different person.

"My pulmonary doctor had called and asked if I would like to take part in a study for an implant for oxygen. I was over the moon with excitement. The thought of nothing on my ears, and no nose-hose was a dream come true. Just to show everything does not go smoothly every time, I had a small problem in surgery, and they had to insert a second catheter that worked just fine. At this point I was no loner part of the study, and I seemed to have fallen through the cracks. My doctor had gone on

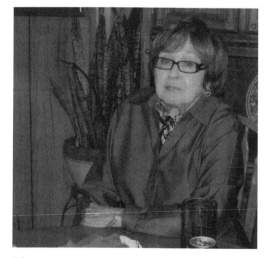

Sherry

maternity leave, so I took matters into my own hands. I found Transtracheal Systems on the Internet. I phoned and was referred me to a pulmonary fellow who introduced me to Dr. Robert Miller at Vanderbilt Hospital. He is always on the cutting edge and sharp as a tack. Through his care and guidance I have had no hospitalizations. Since the TTO was put in back in 1988, I feel I have been blessed to have Dr. Miller as my pulmonary specialist. His is simply the greatest.

"This small catheter has given me a life. I can taste and smell again. My energy is higher, I sleep much better, my color is good, and I no longer "look sick." I now have my femininity back. I wear lipstick and can kiss once again. I simply cannot imagine life without my "SCOOP."

Patient Number 2

Keene is a 59-year-old gentleman who lives just north and west of Denver, Colorado. Keene's introduction to transtracheal oxygen therapy was a bit unique. Keene never had an actual TTO procedure. He had a TTO catheter placed in a standard tracheostomy tube. This is done quite frequently in patients who are weaning from long-term mechanical ventilation. Keene's story picks up in 2002:

"I have used transtracheal oxygen since December 2002 and never did have to wear a nasal cannula for any length of time. In the beginning, I used a standard trach tube with supplemental oxygen. Over time, my trach tube was "downsized" and I was able to remove the trach tube and begin standard SCOOP transtracheal therapy.

"The obvious benefits of the SCOOP catheter are numerous. The nose and ear irritation is totally removed and non-existent. The patient's liter flow should decrease by as much as 50% depending on the patient. The social issue also removed

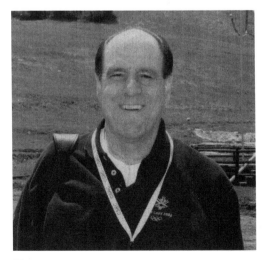

Keene

for the patient and/or family. Cleaning the SCOOP catheter is simple and easy and with a little practice can be done by patients rather quickly.

"The hidden benefits of TTO are all around better health as far as the patient is concerned. The patient feels better due to more efficient oxygen delivery, easier cleaning, removal of any social stigmas, increased patient activity, and just a felling of freedom, that life as it once was….is back.

"Patient to patient conversations take place every day around the country. As I talk to TTO patients one point is made clear, those patients would *never* go back to oxygen delivery using a nasal cannula. On the other hand, it is extremely exciting to talk with prospective transtracheal users. As they listen to all the benefits one question always comes up. That question is "What is the down side of SCOOP transtracheal oxygen therapy? The only answer to that important question is…none for me!

"Let me be clear, each patient is different and therefore circumstances from patient to patient may be different. But from my 7-year experience, there simply is no downside to using transtracheal oxygen therapy. Usually patients are very adaptive to their own situation and tend to overcome any negative. The SCOOP catheter just makes things easier to do. The overall objective is to improve the patient's quality of life. For me, and thousands of patients around the country and world, transtracheal oxygen delivery increases both the *quantity* and *quality* of life."

Patient Number 3

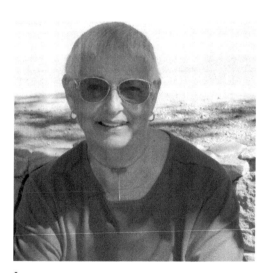

Joanne

Joann is a 73-year-old SCOOP patient who lives in northern New Mexico. Joann has been a SCOOP patient since September 1996. She had been on supplemental nasal oxygen intermittently since the late 1980's. Additionally, Joann is a registered nurse, and so is uniquely qualified to describe her life and use of transtracheal oxygen therapy:

"While working as a nurse in the late 1980's I began to have significant shortness of breath. True to the health care professional stereotype I tried to ignore the blue lips, low oxygen saturations, and extreme fatigue. Finally, my body had taken all it could take and I ended up one shift as the patient in the emergency room. The diagnosis was congestive heart failure (CHF) and Pickwickian Syndrome secondary to a significant weight problem. My life on supplemental oxygen had begun.

"I began a carefully coordinated medical program to lose weight and increase my activity level. It took about 9 months, but I attained my goals and was able to discontinue the oxygen. I hated every minute of the 9 months I had to wear a nasal cannula. My nose was dry and bled often. The tops of my ears were sore, and I was often yanked abruptly when the tubing got hung up on furniture, or accidently stepped on.

"In 1995 I became very symptomatic again and this time I ended up with a diagnosis of secondary pulmonary hypertension. I now knew I would be on oxygen 24/7 for the rest of my life. This was a difficult concept to absorb with all the restrictions this would involve in simple activities of daily living. Then there were the physical and psychological aspects about how I looked and felt about the nasal cannula.

"Somewhere along the line my doctor mentioned the transtracheal catheter as an option. Although my husband George didn't like the idea, I thought it sounded like a much better way to proceed. Thirteen years ago TTO was a simple office procedure. I understand it is now procedure that is done in the hospital's operating room. As with any new skill, it takes some practice and experience to master cleaning techniques. That didn't take so long, and currently I can remove and reinsert the catheter without even looking in the mirror.

"Although I realize a transtracheal oxygen catheter is certainly not for everyone, I can't say enough about the vast increase in so many positive ways compared to the nasal cannula. I've been able to say farewell to sore ears and nosebleeds. My quality of life is enhanced by a very active travel schedule. I have enjoyed several cruises, trips out of town to visit family (especially those grandchildren), and the ability to volunteer with the visiting nurses hospice care and help with the hospital's auxiliary program.

"And so it goes. I am so grateful that the SCOOP was developed a few years before my unplanned need for it. It is a wonderful system of quality materials and engineering for as worry free as possible oxygen delivery system."

Patient Number 4

Nick is a 74 year old Navy veteran of the Second World War now living in Florida. Although he has been a SCOOP patient less than one year, Nick is an example of the perfect candidate for this therapy. Nick's story begins on a road trip to the Grand Canyon:

"In May of 2008 I took a road trip to California, including a stop at the Grand Canyon. After I arrived back in Florida following the road trip my breathing was labored so I contacted my pulmonologist. A six-minute walk test determined that my O2 requirements had increased from 2 L/min at rest to 3 1/2 and from 4 L/min to 6 L/min under effort. That is when my pulmonologist suggested transtracheal oxygen therapy might allow me to continue my very active lifestyle. It didn't sound too good to me initially, but I promised to look into it and did so. I spoke with some TTO2 users, and other experts in the field. Before long I was sold on the on the idea of "giving it a shot."

"In August I informed my pulmonologist that I was interested and would like to pursue getting the procedure done. Together we searched to find a local surgeon who knew how to perform the procedure. From Tampa

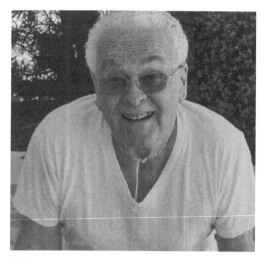

to Orlando to Gainesville, we could not find a surgeon in the surrounding area. I was just two days away from driving all the way up to Johns Hopkins in Baltimore, when I received a call from my pulmonologist stating that he had found a local surgeon who was willing to perform the procedure.

"On May 4th at 1:00 PM, I was in the operating room at The Villages Hospital, and by 9:00am on the 5th, I was on

Nick

TTO2 therapy with a 96% saturation on 1 L/min. At 10:00am on the 6th, I was giving a presentation on COPD, along with my pulmonologist.

"Now I am again "cooking with gas." I have started walking again at 5:00 am on 3 L/min and have completed my six weeks of pulmonary rehab. I am back on the golf course at least once a week (sometimes twice) at 2 L/min. Daily, people are mentioning how strong my voice sounds now. My wife, Jan agrees with them and generally adds that it is also incessant. After having been on the nasal cannula since 2001, I find that I no longer gasp and no longer have sinusitis. My life is so much more "comfortable." The SCOOP catheter is working out beautifully. I am thrilled to be a part of the TTO2 circle of friends and truly hope that many others will join us and get the positive results I have experienced."

1. Richards DW, Barach AL. The effects of oxygen treatment on long periods in patients with pulmonary fibrosis. Amer Rev. Tuberculosis. 1932;26:253-260

2. Richards DW, Barach AL. Prolonged residence in high oxygen atmospheres: Effects on normal individuals and patients with chronic cardiac and pulmonary Insufficiency. Quart J. Med 1934;27:437-66.

3. Petty TL, Finigan MM. The clinical evaluation of prolonged ambulatory oxygen in chronic airway obstruction. Am J Med 1968;45:242-252

4. Roberts SD. Cost Effective oxygen therapy. Ann. Int. Med. 1980:499-500.

5. Nocturnal Oxygen Therapy Trial Group. Continuous or nocturnal oxygen therapy in hypoxemic chronic obstructive disease. Ann. Int. Med. 1980;93: 391-98.

6. Heimlich HJ. Respiratory rehabilitation with a transtracheal oxygen system. Ann. Oto. Rhino. Laryngo. 1982;91:643-47.

7. Christopher KL, Spofford BS, Goodman JR. A program for transtracheal oxygen delivery, assessment of safety and efficacy. Ann Int. Med. Dec. 1987; 6:802-08.

8. Bloom BS et al. Transtracheal portable oxygen in chronic pulmonary disease. (Abstract) Amer. Rev. Resp. Dis. 1985;113:A112.

9. Leger P et al. Transtracheal catheter for oxygen therapy of patients requiring high flows. (Abstract) Respiration 1984;46 (Supplement 1).

10. Banner NR, Govan JR. Long term transtracheal delivery through a microcatheter in patients with hypoxemia due to chronic airways disease. Br. Med. J. 1986;293:111-14.

11. Clifford D, Mender J. Transtracheal oxygen improves survival and reduces hospital costs. (Abstract) 1995;April 151(4):A681.

Chapter 8

My Personal Marathon

Roxlyn G. Cole

Valentine's Day 2003 was my "Delivery Day" for a fountain of life and energy. Not a box of chocolates, but far better — supplemental oxygen. Of course, at first I wasn't so cheery about it. It took almost two years to go through the roller coaster of emotions, including the normal reaction of getting very depressed because I had this COPD disease which required supplemental oxygen. There are stages you go through, and I hit all of them, hard. Now, after six-plus years, I have a much different perspective. I learned to make hard choices to hold my progressive disease at bay and now I feel wonderful.

Being diagnosed with bullous emphysema, even at the mild-borderline moderate stage, including a diffusion problem, makes for an extra challenge when living at higher altitudes. I require oxygen 24/7 here in Littleton, CO, where the elevation is 5500 ft. Altitude decreases one's ability to absorb oxygen from the air. The barometric pressure is less at altitude than at sea level causing the oxygen tension and saturation in the blood to be decreased, even in normal people. At sea level, while sitting, I can have 98% blood oxygen saturations (sats), but at my home at rest it was around 88-90% and much less at exercise. Way too low.

In the beginning

Blood pressure spiking was how my "problem" began. This led to hypertension medicines, along with a stress test that screamed, "pulmonary problems." It seems I had been hypoxic for a pretty long time and was gradually getting worse over the years, moving less, using muscles less — all of which causes a downward spiral in fitness. Everything seemed harder to do. I thought it was my age, or perhaps tiredness from renovating a new home. I was so brain-dim I didn't think that napping and sleeping my days away for over a year was too long a recovery period for some physical exertion. Later I learned I also had mild sleep apnea, for which I now use a CPAP mask at night.

To think I was caught early in the disease only because I finally spoke up and allowed that my chest ached sometimes was my lucky break — that called for a stress test. After the treadmill stress test came an echocardio-gram, a CT, and a full pulmonary function test (PFT). Bless that last test, which discovered the diffusion (DLCO) problem. Simple spirometry showed nothing wrong with me. I try to view all this as a very educational experience. A positive attitude helps.

Taking the first step

My "personal marathon" began with pulmonary rehabilitation classes. They were meant to help me get back to a better level of fitness, since my level of conditioning had deteriorated dreadfully. I was as weak as a kitten.

A personal marathon might begin with five steps, five minutes, or five miles. At the time, any distance seems like a marathon, but you have to do whatever it takes to do a little better than what you are currently doing. This is the first goal in rehab, and it feels similar in difficulty to training for a marathon. It is hard to do. But I wanted to get back to normal. For me, that meant walking more than 15 minutes, and at a brisk, three miles per hour pace. You really have to want to do what it takes.

The nurse who led my pulmonary rehab class told us in the first class the "bad news" of how we would suffocate horribly to death due to our COPD. Tears welled up in almost everyone's eyes, and one gal asked a quavering question, "What is the good news?"

"Oh," she flippantly replied, "they will give you morphine so you won't feel it." At that point I was watching her closely; she was just using a 2x4 to get our attention. After a long pregnant pause, she said, "You can exercise to slow the progress of the disease." She scared the group, and two folks did drop out of class.

Pulse oximeter enters the picture

My husband, a 20-year Navy pilot who was familiar with using supplemental oxygen when flying, said I should get an oximeter since I have a type of COPD in which I don't "feel SOB"; that "short of breath" feeling only came to me with sustained exertion. I needed to check my oxygen sats frequently to see if I was in a safe zone.

The RN discouraged my having my own oximeter because it is "addictive." I ignored her, since that is one of the tools the professionals use. Dammit, I could learn to use it too.

Patients learn how to use thermometers, or how to do their own blood tests to check for insulin needs. We are not stupid. After I did bring the oximeter to class the rehab nurse pretty much ignored me. But it helped me learn to recognize subtle signs that indicated my sats were dropping. My legs would hurt, and I would just feel it was getting difficult and I wanted to sit down. Sure enough, by checking the oximeter any time I started to think "hard to do," I would be in the mid 80% level of blood oxygen saturation.

All of this taught me that some professionals need to update their own knowledge on new rehab techniques and practices. One must be his or her own advocate, learn more, and question even some of the doctors, nurses, and respiratory therapists, as they may need a bit of re-education themselves. Many in that field continue on with the older ways they learned; information which is still in textbooks. We all need to "update" in something.

My oxygen prescription

When the educational part and rehab classes in the gym were completed, I did achieve my first personal goal of a half hour of walking at a little over two miles per hour. I felt it wasn't "good enough." I knew I could do more now with the knowledge learned in the rehab program.

To her credit, the nurse did give me a good start, and did turn me on to liquid oxygen (LOX). I will be forever grateful for that, and actually I can thank her because her blunt force introduction to COPD worked on me. My reaction was to improve above and beyond expectations.

Today I use a liquid portable system with pulse dosing at 2 to 5 liters and for sleep I use 2 liters from my liquid reservoir with my CPAP.

It is the oximeter that has helped me to do extremely well in my own recovery program and to improve my quality of life and functioning. This wonderful little tool tells me if my sats are up or down. It is reassuring if they are good — or informative if they are bad — and I learned to either turn up the oxygen or slow down. I chose to turn my supplemental oxygen flow up above what is considered an adequate level. Adequate, being 92%, isn't good enough for me; all I could do at that O_2 saturation level was sit around. I decided to try different medications since the first inhalers given to me seemed ineffective. For me oxygen works the best, but find out what works for you.

Life-changing experience

With the help of my oxygen, I kept moving at home, learning on the Internet, and reading respiratory magazines. Online I learned to check for reliable information and to always consider the testing group size and check the document date. Words such as "might," "maybe," and "sometimes" could mean the opposite happens. For example, when you read, "Average of five years of life after diagnosis," you have to realize the key word is *average*. If you aren't hanging over an open cooking fire and are getting medical attention and following your doctor's orders, you will not be "average," so don't panic.

Meeting others in the same boat helps too. I got involved in the pulmonary community, attending American Lung Association (ALA) seminars on "How to live with COPD." I also learned about the National Emphysema/COPD Association (NECA), and that led to attendance at their yearly education programs. I joined the group as a "patient advisor."

Then, because another NECA member was otherwise engaged, I gained the profound, life-changing opportunity to attend the four-day Long Term Oxygen Therapy Conference for professionals run by the late Dr. Thomas L. Petty in 2005. Thirteen patients attended, along with more than 100 top doctors, respiratory therapists, and manufacturers of medical equipment. These were all very special people working towards the goal of helping patients with respiratory problems.

I will never forget when Dr. Brian Tiep responded to my comment as to what I do. I said I was "just a patient." He responded in this manner: "*Just?* You are important; patients like you are why we are all here, to learn how we can help you do better." Oh, if only all professionals understood how much their encouragement skyrockets our resolve to try, and how grateful we are to all of them.

It is possible

It was from Dr. Tom Petty that I learned more about the oximeter, and his wish that every patient could have one to "Titrate as you Migrate." *"Titrate as You Migrate"* is a free download from http://www.perf2ndwind.org/html/tompetty/2006/Nov-2006.html. I met the co-authors of his book, *Essentials of Pulmonary Rehab*, the above mentioned Brian Tiep, MD, and Mary Burns, BS, RN.

It was Mary Burns' presentation at that conference that showed me I could walk a lot more. She had a video of a 70-year-old woman training to walk a 10K with her family. I had thought that would never be possible, but because of her, I could at least try to do it; after all, I was only 67.

The additional icing on the cake was meeting Dr. Richard Casaburi of Los Angeles, California. He sat right in front of me, and one of his research papers was on supplemental oxygen used during exercise. He had patients and healthy people breathing air while bicycling in a lab setting. They did not know whether they were breathing normal air or more supplemented oxygenated air. He proved extra oxygen helped even those who were not patients. They improved their exercise capacity, endurance, and speed using supplemental oxygen. It also made for a faster recovery afterward, shortening the aches and pains.

That was all I needed: to be told "it is possible" to do more. I determined to emulate that test, so I asked my online RRT, Mark Mangus, how high a flow was safe. He said the oxygen I could get from my home O_2 systems would not hurt me, and to double check with my own pulmonary specialist to see what equipment I needed to work harder.

My doctor helped by giving me a prescription for higher flows of 7-10 lpm with exercise. Wow, did it help! And Apria Home Healthcare came through for me. They delivered a concentrator that delivered up to 10 lpm, plus a couple of liquid high flow oxygen portables that deliver constant flow

O_2 from 1 lpm up to 15 lpm. They also gave me some compressed gas O_2 cylinders to keep in my car for back up. They and other manufacturers' representatives gave me such encouragement and praise for my efforts to do more. They may not realize it, but these reps helped me as much as the medical teams. Every kind word cheered me on, especially those cheers from some severe stage patients. I was thanked for showing "it is possible" to do more.

The difficult part of all this is trying to train the brain to think positive, and to say "I think I can." The more you do, the more you can do. Keep going and avoid slipping into a downhill spiral. That fear keeps me motivated to "stay on my feet." I have slacked off for a few days to a week, and have found that, oh oh, you lose fitness fast. You must take responsibility for your care and needs.

Getting in the race

While I was still in the pulmonary rehab program, the ALA had a fundraiser 5K run for normal folks and a 1K (6/10th mile) for the lung chal-

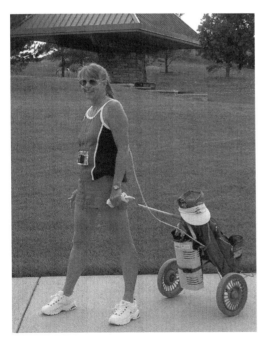

lenged patients. Our rehab group all attended and raised $17,000. It was my first ever "running" event. That walk turned me on to participating in local events. All ages and speeds allowed. Open air, lively friendly people exuding health. I was inspired after the 1K lung challenge walk in 2003, and vowed to do a 5K (3.1 miles) in 2004.

Before getting the high flow liquid oxygen (LOX) portables, my husband learned about a little gizmo called a "wye" — pronounced Y. It looks just like a Y of tubes, and it can be used to connect two or more oxygen

Roxlyn Cole

sources together to produce a higher flow of oxygen. Then we learned higher than 6 lpm required special high flow cannulas and high flow humidifier bottles. We experimented, connecting/combining the concentrator, E tanks, and LOX tanks until I had a good setup rigged to sit next to the treadmill where I could keep walking as long as I wanted and was able to turn up the flow knobs as needed without interruption. (Editorial Note (LN): This should only be done with professional advice. For patients encouraged by Lyn's activity, we strongly recommend that you review this with your medical team before trying it.)

For walking outdoors, an old golf bag cart worked great for carrying one high flow tank, which would last me around an hour, but two or more tanks? With a 10K (6.2 miles) as my next goal, just how would I carry enough oxygen for the time it would take for that long of a walk?

Just by odd chance, I spotted a baby jogger stroller as we drove by a consignment shop. It was out on the grass along with others to attract attention. The light bulb turned on in my brain. That was exactly what I needed to transport four liquid oxygen tanks, a back-up of compressed oxygen gas, and water, oximeter, cell phone, wind breaker, and any other needs for a four hour walk. I use the Caire High Flow oxygen capable of up to 15 liters flow for intense exercise.

This began my passion for solving oxygen problems, what to use, and how to deal with it all. I learned which systems worked well for me for exercise and which for plain old "living" at a slower pace.

Enter TTO

Next problem: how could I use less oxygen, perhaps fewer tanks? Bingo! Try out the transtracheal oxygen system (TTO). (*See Chapter 7*)

Dr. Tom Petty named my story about that, "Necking with Oxygen," which appeared in *Everything Respiratory*. After three-plus years of the irritating soreness of the nose hose cannula, I opted to have a Fast Tract TTO placed in my trachea, with the encouragement of John Goodman, BS, RRT.

I had no idea it would be so wonderful. It did cut my oxygen needs in half for slower activities and somewhat for exercise. It made breathing easier, and I got my face back, which was nicer than I had imagined. No more need to take a cannula off to blow my nose or wash my face. No more bloody noses or pressure lines. And the oxygen delivery tubes were more discreet under my shirt. Even medical personnel didn't notice it — even when I left it open and uncovered. I absolutely love what the SCOOP TTO does for me. (To learn more about transtracheal oxygen go to their web site: www.tto2.com or call 1-800-527-2667.) *(See Chapter 7)*

I also learned more about starting my own personal exercise program from Mary Burns' program and read "The Essentials of Pulmonary Rehabilitation." (Editorial note: A few copies of this booklet are still available.) It is so sad there aren't enough rehabilitation centers located nearby for all lung challenged patients, and I believe the educational part of that program would help even the most mild COPD patients learn what is ahead for them, to see all stages of disease in the other participants. This made a profound impression upon me. I did not want to get worse. It might help some to take charge of their lives and to try harder to quit smoking and to make good choices to feel and function better.

In Denver, the ALA had a COPD Summit and extended invitations to medical professionals and patients, and they began a COPD coalition to build a program for Colorado COPD patient needs. *(See Chapter 13)* It was wonderful sitting in with the research section. I learned so much, and contributed from the patient's point of view.

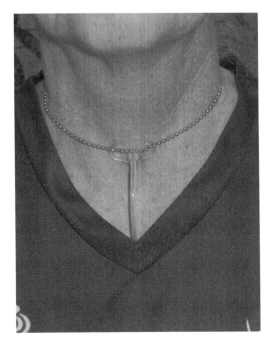

Necking with Oxygen; a Fast Tract TTO

Stay inspired

In 2004 I walked not only a 10K, but my first half marathon. Two half marathons followed in 2005, and since then I've been walking up to three a year. That 13.1 miles is enough for me, although I tentatively speculated on trying a full marathon.

But at age 71, I decided I have gone far enough and will leave that to the younger folks. Maybe it is burnout. One has to stay inspired to keep moving. Music is my biggest helper. One can listen to book tapes, watch TV, and even read when going slowly on the treadmill. The TV distracts me while lifting small weights and using ankle weights for leg work. Resistance moves and stretches all have a lot of benefit to the body. Yoga, tai chi, plain old dancing with a partner, or holding onto a chair for balance helps many people as well. Sing, dance, play a wind instrument; any sustained activity will be of benefit and then a little more.

Although you do have to adjust the amount of moving you can do to your individual stage in COPD, I have been told, "any age, any stage," will benefit from exercise. Walking a half marathon is way beyond what is necessary for improving one's function and fitness. You can call me an exercise addict; it is just my idea of "fun."

Even small moves pay off

A great ultimate goal, or "personal" marathon for anyone is to do a half hour a day, slowly working up to walking at 20-25 minutes per mile. Once at that level, extend your endurance after the walk with your own choice of fun activities, which might include family, home chores and maintenance, food shopping, and socializing. It all adds up to making travel easier. You gain the endurance to keep moving.

Once you work through that "SOB" and get comfortable with it, moving does truly get easier. If you cannot walk because of other limitations you can move in other ways to build muscles and achieve an aerobic activity. Ask your doctor for a program of exercises that applies to you. Then try and try again, and you will not regret the effort. Benefits are proportional to what you put into it. First learn, and then *do*.

Encouragement is key

COPD ALERT is where I met Mike McBride. *(See Chapter 9)* I was talking about the ALA's stair climb fundraiser. He popped in and said he was from the Denver area, and he wanted to join my COPDers+ team. He had climbed 14,000 ft. mountains.

The 47 flights that year weren't enough; he went on to climb the Hancock in Chicago, and then to complete the full Boston Marathon in 2009. Now even *that* marathon is possible with COPD, pulling a cart with tanks of oxygen.

Mike has been a huge help, telling me I could do a 10K and then a half marathon. Friends and support groups all are a great source of encouragement. Find out what you want to know and how to manage your disease. But above all, *move* towards formal exercise.

Roxlyn Cole's tips for people with COPD

Seek out "how to" information, if not on the computer, at the library. Or you can call the American Lung Association help line at 1-800-586-4872, the COPD Foundation's answer line at 1-866-316-2673, or the National Jewish Health Lung Line at 1-800-222-5864.

Ask your oxygen provider for manuals on your equipment. Find out, learn, and improve. Look for educational handout materials in your doctor's office or in hospital waiting areas. Subscribe to respiratory related magazines.

Everything Respiratory is a magazine that almost makes reading about lung challenges fun. It is inspirational and informative in language a patient can understand, and it has many patients' stories. Cost is about $14.99 for four issues per year. Ordering information: www.ERmag.org, 877-376-2448.

COPD DIGEST FREE is available at http://www.copddigest.org/ or by calling the COPD Information Line at 1-866-316-COPD (2673). Ask for a subscription and the other free information packets.

The National Home Oxygen Patient Association publishes a monthly newsletter with timely information regarding association activities, health and travel tips, and ways to communicate with other oxygen users. Membership in the organization is around $15.00; call 1-888-646-7244 or go to:
http://www.homeoxygen.org/member.html to join.

The Pulmonary Paper costs circa $15.00 and includes 6 issues: http://www.pulmonarypaper.org/. 1-800-950-3698.

Check COPD support websites for some interesting and vital information. I was thrilled to be listed on the main page of COPD ALERT, www.copd-alert.com, along with my beginning story, which was published in the COPD Digest: http://www.copd-alert.com/LynCole.pdf

I spend time writing what I hope are inspirational and helpful stories for magazines and on my COPD information blog: http://profiles.yahoo.com/roxlyngcd.

Check other groups online, and local Better Breathers. Talk, learn, live.

Lastly, keep trying, even if only for a one second increase per day. It all adds up, and it really works. My pulmonary function numbers have remained constant for six-plus years now, except for the normal aging factor. Keep learning and keep moving any way you can.

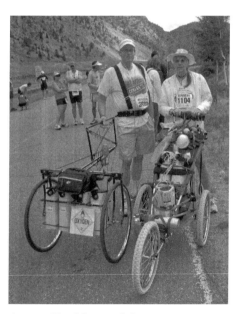

A pair of healthy oxyphiles

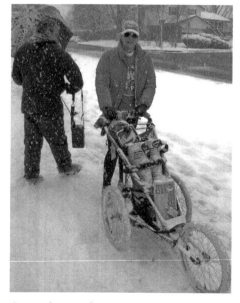

Snowy lungs a la carte

Chapter 9

Miles, Mountains and Stairs, Oh My!

Michael McBride

My adventures as an oxy-phile began in 2005. I was no stranger to COPD, as my mother had been battling the disease for several years, but I never thought it would happen to me.

As 2004 was coming to a close, it looked like 2005 was going to be a banner year. My only daughter was expecting my first grandchild. Unfortunately, this happiness was tainted. Christmas 2004, Mom had a flair-up of her COPD. By the first week of the new year, she was readmitted with yet another exacerbation, and roughly a week later, she was sent home with the grim prognosis that there was nothing left they could do. This devastating news cast a pall over the excitement of the upcoming birth.

My granddaughter, Haley, arrived on January 27 to a joyous family. Sadly, mom passed away ten days later on the night before her 52nd wedding anniversary. The funeral was held the following week. It was a stressful time, with the joy of Haley's arrival and the sadness of mom's passing.

I had been short of breath all week long. I do have other medical issues, but this was alarming. I would go halfway up a flight of stairs, then stop to catch my breath. The post-funeral reception was held in the basement of the First Methodist Church in Golden, CO. A wheelchair ramp stretches from the basement to street level. I had to stop twice walking up that ramp to go home.

The day after the funeral I had an appointment at University Hospital in Denver for another condition. That is when my life changed forever. What I had thought was an irritating shortness of breath was far more severe. The doctors ordered x-rays that revealed I had what appeared to be pneumonia in four of five lobes. They immediately scheduled a CT scan and released me with a portable oxygen tank and orders to return within an hour and a half. They told me to go home and collect some things for a hospital stay. If I wasn't back by that time, they would call the police!

I got home, packed a few things, called my significant other, Cameron, and headed back to the hospital. Thus began my life as an oxy-phile.

The diagnosis and further complications

Once back at the hospital, I was placed in a negative pressure isolation room. The next thing I knew everyone coming in the room was decked out in moon suits — gowns, masks, gloves — the whole nine yards. The reason for this was they thought I had tuberculosis. I told them that there was no way I had tuberculosis but I couldn't change their minds. They were convinced I had TB, so I was going to remain encased in the negative pressure isolation room until the tests results confirmed I was right.

Normally, I wouldn't be too concerned, but I had some important plans in the works. This was Wednesday, and Haley's baptism brunch was scheduled for Sunday. Cameron and I were planning to host 60 people at our house.

It takes three days to cultivate the TB culture and I would not be released until the test results were confirmed. In order not to waste time, the doctors started pumping me full of antibiotics to kill the pneumonia. By Saturday, it was obvious I was going to miss my granddaughter's baptism. I was spiking a fever and the x-rays showed that even after the doses of antibiotics, there was something growing in my lungs.

Sunday was one of the lowest days of my life. I was trapped in a hospital isolation room, missing an event I had waited my lifetime for, and the doctors did not have a definitive answer for what was wrong with me! There is no way to convey just how upset and frustrated I was.

I started the next week with a biopsy. Since the TB results were negative, they thought I might have cancer. My x-rays were clearing up, my fever had subsided, and sputum tests showed no signs of bacteria. The biopsy was a mixed result. It showed that I didn't have cancer, but I had bronchiolitis obliterans organizing pneumonia, or BOOP. Funny name, terrible diagnosis.

The short version is that I had garden-variety pneumonia and my immune system geared up to fight the infection, which is what normally happens. However, in my case, I was given antibiotics to take care of the infection, but my immune system did not back off. Instead, it continued to attack the area where the infection had been. Instead of helping, my immune system was damaging my lungs further. I couldn't believe it! My own body was attacking the most vulnerable organ in my body, my lungs!

It took a week and a half to make the diagnosis of emphysema/COPD and determine that my bacterial pneumonia had been complicated by bronchial obliterans (BOOP). When I entered the hospital, I was a long-time smoker. When I left eight days later, I was a non-smoker. When I returned two weeks after that I was told that when I was previously admitted, they were not sure if I was going to make it through the night! Yikes! I had too much to live for!

A history of exercise helps

When Cameron returned to college in 1992, we needed a quiet house so he could study. I used the time to create a relatively formal workout schedule. At the time, we lived in a condominium complex, complete with a racquet club and extensive gym for residents' use.

I was one of those strange animals who would workout three to four times a week, and smoke on the way home. When I was at the hospital, I was told that the only thing that I could do to slow down or potentially stop the progression of my disease was to exercise. It was my discipline of going to the gym on a regular basis, coupled with the heartfelt desire that Haley have time with her grandfather, which prepared me to assume my role as a certified oxy-phile.

Initially, I was sent home with oxygen to be worn 24/7 until I had fully recovered from the BOOP and pneumonia. I was to use 1-1.5 liters at rest and 2 liters at night. It was recommended that I get an oximeter to monitor my saturation levels and to keep track of them in a note book.

Adventure No. 1: Logging the miles

I began my walking career while still an inpatient. I was on the 4th floor and I began walking the hallways. I counted tiles on the floor, and figured out how many laps it would take to make a mile.

Once home, I walked every day. My first outing was about six blocks. I was so tired that I thought I would not make it home. But I kept after it. I drove through my neighborhood, marking out a 3.4 mile route that began and ended at home. It took me just over a month, but I completed my first lap.

Although I enjoyed the exercise, I needed something to strive for. I set my sights on walking the annual Bolder Boulder 10K race. The Boulder, CO, tradition attracts large crowds and is run on Memorial Day.

In 2005, there were just over 46,000 runners and walkers. Knowing I needed to tote my own oxygen, I brought a Caire Stroller to Recreational Equipment Inc. (REI) and asked a sales person to help me find a backpack I could race in. On race day, I secured my oxygen in my new backpack and pinned bib number 7475 on my red shirt. I jumped onto a shuttle bus at 6 a.m. to hang out with 46,000 athletes. The race starts in waves set by estimated finishing time. I was in one of the later waves, so I found my corral and cooled my heels, taking in the sights for an hour and a half before my wave got its start.

Setting the pace

The Bolder Boulder begins at the north end of Boulder and ends at University of Colorado's Folsom Field toward the south end of the city. Racers have to be inside the stadium on the metal covered track surrounding the football field by a certain time or you miss the Memorial Day festivities.

The Citizen's Race starts before the Elite Race, so everyone has a chance to be in the stadium to watch the invited international speedsters fly across the finish line. I wasn't sure if I could make it to the stadium in time. I followed a woman who set a rigorous pace for me. As we crossed the finish line, I thanked her for being my pacesetter.

With tears in her eyes, she said, "I had to lose 98 pounds just so I could do this race." I held up my cannula and commented, "I had a few obstacles this past year myself."

Upping the ante

I decided 2006 was the year I would take my walking in race events to new heights. My first race of the season was the five-mile Cherry Creek

Sneak (CCS), a popular race through the upscale Cherry Creek Shopping district. From there I did my second Bolder Boulder in May, and I tackled the inaugural Colorado Colfax Marathon and Half-Marathon in June, doing the 13.1 mile race.

The warm day found me pushing my oxygen in a baby stroller. Most people did not quite know what to think about me. I must have been quite a sight. They could not see what was in the stroller, and many of the volunteer course marshals tried to enforce the rules, stating that I could not push my "baby" in the race.

My "babies" were made of hard plastic and it should have been obvious that I was not their Dad! It took my buddy Teri and me 3 hours and 59 minutes to complete 13.1 miles. That is averaging an 18.15-minute mile.

All downhill

Bitten by the half marathon bug, I found another one. The Slacker Half Marathon is an annual race held in Georgetown, which is in the mountains. Starting at Loveland Basin Ski area, which is 10,600 feet above sea level, the Slacker descends to 8,500 feet, returning us to Georgetown.

Without a doubt, the Slacker is the hardest race on my schedule. The first five miles are on a dirt road that is really a U.S. Forest Service emergency access road, meaning it is not a "groomed" road by any stretch of the imagination. If you think going downhill is easier, it can be very deceiving. Going 13.1 miles downhill is punishing to your legs and feet. That being said, I love this race; the scenery is spectacular and the area peaceful beyond belief.

Las Vegas Marathon

Now that I knew I could complete a half marathon in 3.5 hours, I wanted to step it up a notch and try a full marathon. I found out the Las Vegas Marathon kept the course open until everyone finished, and better still, I learned there would be a fellow COPD athlete in the area.

I had been sharing emails with Roxlyn "Lyn" Cole (*see Chapter* 8) since the fall of 2005. It turns out that the American Association for Respiratory Care was having its annual convention in Las Vegas, starting the

Monday following the race. Lyn and her husband Lou were going to be in Las Vegas to help the publisher of Everything Respiratory magazine, Holly Lockwood, and they would be attending the convention. I had been able to talk my good friend, Mary Ann, into coming to the race to help me, so I had a 3-person pit crew to follow me in a car and help me swap out the liquid oxygen every two hours or so throughout the race.

At one point, the cannula froze so hard that it shattered like glass when I pulled it off the tank. Not good! I was not last in that race, but close. My feet hurt so badly I could barely walk. But it was worth every moment of pain.

Exacerbation gets in the way

After completing the Las Vegas Marathon, I decided that I would try to do a marathon each year, and my 2007 choice was going to be the Oklahoma City Memorial Marathon.

The race was being held on Sunday, April 29, and we had made plans to drive from Denver to Oklahoma City. On Wednesday, April 19, I called my pulmonologist. I told him I was not feeling well, but since I had a race to get to, asked if he could prescribe a course of medication to deal with it. Like a true race addict, I did not want to miss a race I was looking forward to and had trained for.

Big mistake! I felt crummy through the weekend and by Tuesday afternoon found myself admitted to Lutheran Hospital with a severe case of pneumonia. I couldn't believe it. Not only was I going to miss my race, but when I was released from the hospital, my oxygen needs doubled. I was now a high-flow oxy-phile!

High flow for me is 4-6 lpm at rest and 10+ when exercising. When walking a marathon my lpm is usually 15-20. My nose gets so dry from the high flow, I battle bloody noses for days afterward.

Race walking

I discovered that there are not a lot of marathons that are walker friendly and the only way I was going to be able to do long distance races was to get faster. There was no way that I could run. My higher oxygen requirements while exercising led me to discover the Olympic sport of race walking.

Race walking allows me to walk faster, while being more efficient. But the increased oxygen demand required me to get creative with my transport system. Lyn Cole uses a baby-jogger baby stroller, but strollers are difficult for me to steer. I turned, again, to a friend.

My buddy, Bill Manley, and I were talking about my troubles with oxygen transportation. I told him I needed something like a cross between a rickshaw and a trailer. We put our heads together, and the "The Cart" would become the solution. The Cart made her debut at the walker friendly Portland Marathon on October 5, 2007.

Cameron accompanied me on the trip, and I was really ready to go and give it my all. But, as luck would have it, we had oxygen equipment problems. The large reservoir valve was frozen open and we lost all my back-up O2. I was not going to finish the race without oxygen. We left the race area and headed back to the motel with the hope of reaching someone at the local Apria office. I was able to maintain my saturation levels above at sea level with pursed lip breathing and staying very calm, but we had mountains to cross before we were back home. Even if I didn't need the oxygen, having it along would make me feel better.

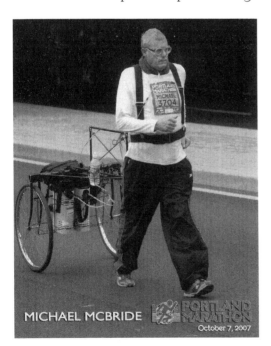

MICHAEL MCBRIDE

2007 Portland Marathon

When we arrived back in Denver, the Denver Marathon was a week away. My shins were hurting, but I wanted to race in the half marathon event. I loaded up on Vicodin, and headed out to the race. This was not a good idea!

The weather was truly rotten. Sleet, snow, and cold! I also learned something about Vicodin. It is a great pain reliever, except when it quits working, and taking more does not help.

I made it halfway through the race and had to call it quits. I hobbled back to the starting line. It was a good thing I stopped. I had stress-fractured both legs.

Getting healthy again

I vowed to get healthy for the 2008 season. I worked out diligently at my local YMCA, prepping for the Oklahoma City Memorial Marathon in April. My real goal was to do well enough to qualify for the Mother of all Marathons — the Boston Marathon.

Oklahoma City was fun. The people were fantastic. The weather started out crummy with sleet and snow, but by the end it was bright sunshine and a bit of wind. And I did what I set out to do. I qualified for Boston.

On to Boston

On April 20, 2009, I became the first person with COPD to enter and complete the Boston Marathon in regulation time: 7 hours 31 minutes 36 seconds, averaging 17.14-minute miles for 26.2 miles. The Boston Marathon is the most amazing spectacle I have ever been a part of. I had the privilege of doing the marathon with Steve Gaudet, a respiratory therapist with severe, end-stage asthma from San Francisco. This man can barely breathe and yet he completed the event a second before me. I am still in awe of that accomplishment.

We started an hour ahead of the field, and were cheered on as the speedy runners passed us. Finishing this historic race humbles me in indescribable ways. I marvel at how much focus I was able to maintain for the 7.5 hours. Heartbreak Hill is everything they say it is. I have climbed steeper hills with my cart, but Heartbreak Hill is actually a combination of six hills located between miles 16 and 21. When I crested the last hill, I honestly do not think I could have withstood another.

Adventure No. 2: Climbing mountains

I am a third generation Colorado native on my mother's side. Although I was raised in Golden, and went to college in Gunnison, it was not until I was diagnosed with COPD that I thought about the mountains around me. Colorado has 54 mountains over 14,000 feet ("14'ers"), and this Colorado native had never climbed any of them. I was determined to change this. The last weekend of September in 2005, my new life as a COPD oxy-phile was about to take another twisting turn.

My buddy Teri told of a place along I-70 that was close to the highway and well maintained. It was Myers Ranch Park, but I did not know the name. I was not having any luck finding Teri's place, but I saw the exit for Mt. Evans.

What the heck? I had never been up this way, and I wasn't even aware that Mt. Evans (14,263 feet) was a 14'er. I paid my entry fee and the park ranger told me that this would be the last weekend the road would be open for the season.

I started about 10:30 a.m., and figured I would be up and down in about three hours. Fortunately, this ascent was done prior to my being a high flow oxy-phile, but, truth be told, I was oxygen deprived most of the climb. The hike is beautiful but it took a lot longer than I thought it would. I would walk about 20 steps, stop, catch my breath, and then take another 20. I had my oximeter and two full 6 liter Caire strollers with me. I had the flow set at 2 liters and at that rate I would have about 5 hours of oxygen. I kept checking the oximeter and I was about 88 on 3 liters so in order to conserve I would walk awhile at 3 then back to 2. I guess knowing what I do now, that was risky business.

As I was nearing the top, I was down to ten step cycles. Those ten steps became five and the scree was getting larger and hard to maneuver over. When I was about level with the parking lot, I had about 80 minutes of oxygen left and made the decision to forego the summit, which would have been about another 30 minutes of walking, and I headed down the road to my truck. I did something I am adamantly opposed to on the way down. There are a series of switchbacks leading to the summit and I went cross-country rather than follow the road. I asked the mountain to forgive my insult and hoped I would get down okay.

Elevation and oxygen deprivation do funny things to your brain. Determining up from down becomes nearly impossible. I was disorientated and ended up turning around and heading back up the mountain. It would have been a disaster had not a couple of bicyclists spotted me and pointed me in the right direction! I did run out of oxygen, but fortunately it was all downhill at that point and I was about a mile away from my pickup. Better still, I could see it off in the distance. I don't recall checking my sats at this point, but I'm certain they were in the low 80s.

Two 14'ers a summer

Despite this rather scary experience, I was hooked on the mountains. Wintertime was spent planning which mountains I could summit and return within the 5.5-6 hours of oxygen I can physically carry in my backpack.

June 2006 found me attempting Gray's Peak. I talked my sister Patty into being my 14'er partner and off we went. We made steady progress, but by about 13,800 feet I was getting tired. Patty was walking ahead of me about 30 feet and I was almost ready to toss in the towel, when all of sudden we came over the crest. The peak was in reach.

What an astounding sight and spiritual experience to be standing at the high point of land for miles around and look down. We took several pictures and then headed down. I was, once again, concerned about not having enough oxygen, and with good reason. I ran out again and it was really slow going at the end. We completed the round-trip in six hours.

In August 2006, Patty and I decided to climb Quandary Peak, a 7-mile roundtrip hike that is extremely steep at the beginning, then levels to about a 10% grade. For the last 800 feet, the rise is at a 60-degree angle.

The weather was overcast with a light mist, but we thought it would not get any worse. It was chilly, but not slippery, until we got to about 13,600 feet.

We met a group of people

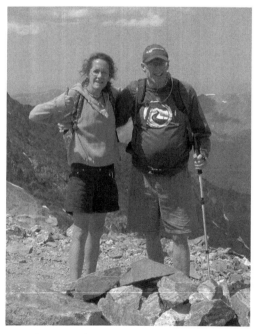

Atop Grays Peak, June 2006, Elevation 14,270 ft.

who seemed to appear out of nowhere at the foot of the cloud cover. They suggested we not go any further because the weather was getting worse. It was the first week of August and ahead of us was rain, snow, thunder, and lightning. We were dressed and prepared for everything except lightening. Just two weeks before, the partner of one of my doctors was struck and killed by lightning while attempting a 14'er.

I looked at my sister and announced, "We're going down, now!"

Even with the extra tank, I ran out of oxygen. Patty hiked down to the truck, picked up my spare tank, and hiked back up. While we did not make it to the summit, it was still a remarkable effort. I had never seen mountain goats in the wild, and a mother and her kid passed within 50 feet of us. That alone was worth the trip.

The rest of my summer was busy, and I was not able to do any more hiking. Then my pneumonia bout in April 2007 not only caused me to graduate up to a high flow liquid oxygen system, but also grounded me from the mountains because I am unable to carry enough oxygen. That was a big part of my reasoning to have the transtracheal procedure done in December 2008.

One of the benefits of having a TTO is reduced oxygen requirements. For me, I have had no reduction at rest (still using 4-6 liters to maintain 94+%) but it has cut my exercise needs by 40%. Where in the past I would require 15-20 lpm, I now use 10-12.

Adventure No. 3: Taking the stairs

I joined the online community COPD-ALERT in May of 2005. Through COPD-ALERT, I learned that Lyn Cole was looking for volunteers to do an ALA stair climbing event in Denver called "Run the Register." The race took place in the Wells Fargo Building, which features a "cash register" type of architecture at its top. Our team was comprised mostly of COPD patients: Lyn Cole, Marilyn Sundt-Quibble, and myself. I climbed all 52 flights, but it was not pretty.

In 2007, I found the "Hustle up the Hancock" in Chicago. This is a 95-floor race, from the basement to the observation level on the 94th floor. On the day of the race, the cloud cover was so low the upper 20 floors were hidden from view. I made a conscious decision not to go up before the race, because I wanted to see the view as a treat for finishing the race. No treat. It was socked in.

In 2008, the Denver race was moved to the Republic Plaza Building with a name change to "Run the Republic." I was able to recruit some new team members for the 56-floor event, and Team COPD+ expanded to 12. In 2009, I entered the inaugural Climb Chicago, which was held at the Presidential Towers, a residential complex located west of downtown Chicago. You climb four buildings for a total of 180 floors. I used a Caire High Flow Stroller in my trusty package for the stair climb. At Chicago's lower elevation, I had the flow set at 8 lpm and that maintained my saturation levels at 95% while my heart rate was hovering between 145-150.

I marched up those 360 flights with a finishing time of 1:06:13. Not only did I accomplish an amazing feat, there were people behind me, so I was not last. I was thrilled to have passed another oxy-phile milestone.

Happy to be an inspiration

Since my diagnosis in 2005, I have completely quit smoking and completed three full marathons, over 20 half marathons, several 10Ks, a couple of 5-milers, and a handful of 5K events toting oxygen on my back, pushing oxygen in front of me, and now pulling oxygen behind me in "The Cart." I have completed several stair climbing events, and I have even climbed mountains. I have met some incredible people along the way, and have a singular goal in every race — crossing the finish line. Getting a nice finisher's medal is not bad either!

All of my adventures as an oxy-phile have been selfish in nature. I did them to test myself, to be alive and moving, and to feel connected to the universe. The fact that people find inspiration in them still amazes me, but if my getting out there inspires just one person to put down the remote and get off the couch, I'll shout "Alleluia" from the highest peak I can get to in Colorado.

"Fishing is not an escape from life, but often a deeper immersion into it..."
— Harry Middleton —

Chapter 10

Coast to Coast on O$_2$

Mark Junge

It was probably decades ago when the idea of a cross-country bicycle trip bubbled up in my brain. If I told you that it all started with my very first bike, I'd be lying. That clunky steel monster, whose brand name I can't remember, had balloon tires and a Bendix coaster brake. It was an antique when I found it rusting in the grass in a neighbor's backyard, and its rehabilitation cost me a summer's wages earned by mowing lawns. My next bike was a Schwinn Varsity that served as transportation while I was in college and until I could afford to buy a car.

The decision to ride across the country on a bicycle was not made by someone who knew exactly what he wanted to do and what steps he had to take to accomplish that goal. I do not have an engineering mentality. Rather, the idea fermented slowly and became a reality due to circumstances.

The goal developed partly from a love of adventure that was embedded in my genes. My mother loved to gamble and my father was like the bear that went over the mountain to see what he could see. My innate wanderlust was fed by antique *National Geographic* magazines my father had found stored in a barn, and by a passel of books about travel and adventure, ranging from Mark Twain's *Tom Sawyer* and *Huckleberry Finn* to Jack Kerouac's *On the Road*. Of course, the "Wizard of Oz" was my favorite film. Like Dorothy, I wanted to follow the yellow brick road to Emerald City. Along the way, I would make new friends and have one adventure after another.

Baby boomers don't quit

A college education offered a good enough reason to travel. At Western State College in the remote Gunnison Valley of Colorado, I was lucky to have history professors who were not only academically astute but also storytellers. Studying history helped me understand causation and how people are products of their generations.

For example, a common trait of the post-World War II baby boomers is that they quit gobbling up life only when they quit breathing. Perhaps that is true of every generation, but the post World War II generation, in particular, was raised in a period of intense scientific and technological expansion. They have an optimistic attitude that nothing is impossible. The sky is the limit. New is exciting. Old is moldy.

When I finally made the decision to cross America on a bike, I knew that it would not be behind a windshield on a trouble-free interstate highway system that the American Society of Civil Engineers has judged to be one of the seven wonders of the United States. Instead, I would be in closer contact with one of the world's seven continents, feeling North America rumbling under my bike tires. I would coast down two-lane country roads under blue skies laced with puffy white clouds, inhaling the aphrodisiac of Mother Earth, and the chemicals of the Industrial Age. The scene would be reminiscent of a Dick and Jane primer, or perhaps a Norman Rockwell illustration for the *Saturday Evening Post*, and I would wave as I rolled past fathers mowing lawns and mothers in aprons hanging the family wash on clotheslines.

The Lincoln Highway

My route of travel would be from west to east along the historic Lincoln Highway. Named for our 16th president, the road was the nation's first transcontinental automobile highway. From Lincoln Park in San Francisco, "America's Main Street" stretches 3,400 miles to Times Square in Manhattan. It crosses the mid-section of America, intersecting five state capitols, dozens of county seats, and nearly 200 congressional districts.

The name Lincoln is everywhere, on streets and avenues, businesses, shopping centers, and parks. For example, in Cheyenne, Wyoming, where I live, Lincolnway is the main east-west route through downtown, and near the intersection of Capitol Avenue and Lincolnway is the Lincoln Theater. Forty miles west of Cheyenne at the highest point along Interstate 80 is the Lincoln Monument. Robert Russin's huge bronze bust of the Great Emancipator gazes downward under beetling brows at the traffic below.

The single ribbon of concrete and asphalt spanning the continent from the Atlantic to the Pacific is no longer America's Main Street binding the country together. Interstate 80 has replaced it. Still, as an historian and a romantic, I envisioned the two-lane Lincoln Highway, flanked by crumbling remnants of a pre-World War II culture, as a nostalgic thoroughfare through America's past, one in which there still might be red brick pavers, concrete S-curve bridges, Burma Shave signs, cantilevered filling stations, motor court cabins, and mom and pop cafes where waitresses in starched aprons served milk shakes and apple pie.

A life-altering event

In the fall of 2002 my dream of a bicycle trip down the yellow-striped Lincoln Highway was blasted into smithereens. A flu-like illness compromised my ability to breathe. What else could go wrong? I had already experienced two open heart surgeries, a hip replacement, and other, minor operations. But this was different. The diagnosis —following a major biopsy in which a piece of my lung was clipped and sent to the Mayo Clinic — was blood clots. How did they get into my lungs? Maybe they came from those previous surgeries. Maybe it was genetic, maybe diet, or both. It didn't matter. The blood clots that clobbered up my lungs also blocked my bicycle plans.

Scarring caused by the blood clots made it difficult for me to catch a breath during any form of exertion except sitting. I needed supplemental oxygen, especially when sleeping. This was more than "a revolting development," as Chester A. Riley used to say. It was more than revolting and it was more than temporary. This disability meant a lifestyle change, not only for me but also for my wife, Ardath.

We had been married for 36 years, had two sons, and in order to help support the family she had worked nearly 30 years as an elementary school teacher. In addition, she had supported me through all my surgeries, and now she would have to support me again.

Ardath is a natural worrier and this situation only antagonized her anxiety. She did not always show her anxiety, but I knew it was inside of her. She realized that the process of growing old together had changed. Mine was not a temporary problem, but one that would be present for the rest of our lives together. Like a majority of people who find out that they need supplemental oxygen, I became depressed and she had to deal with my depression. A cloud now hung over my head but it affected both of our daily lives.

Life goes on

Regardless, I was still a dreamer. I still believed that anything was possible and that progress was inevitable and beneficial. Technology would find a way to make things better. As predictable as the sun coming up in the East every day, someone, somewhere, had a solution for this problem.

Fortunately, in my case the person who held the technological key was Cheyenne pulmonologist, Dr. Laura Brausch. She suggested a major biopsy in order to learn, more specifically, what was wrong with my lungs. Dr. Brausch understood my need to be active. When we found the problem, she prescribed a blood thinner; portable, liquid oxygen; and an oximeter for measuring my blood oxygen saturation. During the daytime I would be on a 1.5 to 2.0 liter per minute flow rate unless I needed more oxygen for everyday tasks, in which case I could turn the knob of my Helios oxygen canister up to the rate of 4 lpm. Those were the technological tools provided by a competent professional. The rest was up to me.

Gradually I came to understand that my lifestyle might not have to change as drastically as I first feared. Using portable oxygen, I went back to the Cheyenne Family YMCA and developed an exercise routine. Very quickly, I discovered that I could push myself to stay in shape. It was simply a matter of obtaining enough oxygen to do it. Amazingly, I found that I could actually lift weights without supplemental oxygen. In fact, during lifting exercises the oximeter showed that my blood oxygen saturation actually increased from 88 up to as high as 94 or 95, depending upon how much concentration I put into breathing. Breath control came from weightlifting training, which taught me to breathe deeply before lifting and exhale deeply while pushing or pulling weights.

Life as I knew it had not come to end. Supplemental oxygen would allow me to exercise. I could work. I could perform up to my own expectations. In addition, best of all, the dream of a cross-country bicycle trip was still alive. It would simply require getting enough air in my lungs . . . and enough money to pay for the trip.

Finding a sponsor

The money was a worry for both Ardath and me. We were in limbo. I had taken early retirement and she was ready to retire after a 30-year teaching career. We were both 59 and it would be three years before we would become eligible for Social Security. I decided to find a sponsor. Bicycle companies were not the answer. They sponsored young champions and teams. Ardath suggested contacting the company that manufactured my Helios portable liquid oxygen system. That was the logical idea, but it had not occurred to me. At that moment, my personal goal of bicycling across America began morphing into something much more altruistic.

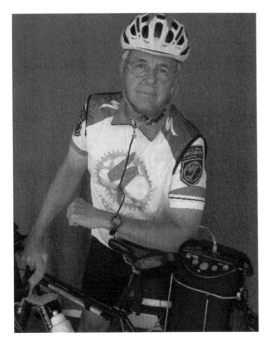

On the back of my Helios liquid oxygen canister was the name of its manufacturer, Nellcor Puritan Bennett, and the parent company, Mallinckrodt. Both, I came to find out, were subsidiaries of Tyco International, a large, multi-faceted corporation. In 2004, I phoned Mallinckrodt's marketing executive officer, Randy Krotz, in St. Louis. Randy listened to my pitch without saying much. Later, when I kidded him about reading his email while I was talking, he told me that the cross-

Mark Junge

country bicycling idea had a certain public relations "bite." Unbeknownst to me, Randy was beginning to formulate a much broader scenario for my escapade than I could imagine.

The Tyco Corporation, Mallinckrodt's parent company, decided to sponsor the bicycle trip. Plans laid by the company posited me as an example of portable oxygen's benefits. Aware of the pressures that would accompany intense media coverage, Randy Krotz asked me, would I be comfortable being a poster boy for COPD and Tyco? At my age, given my previous health problems, I realized that it was now or never. It was not difficult to snap back an answer. Of course, I would be happy to be a spokesperson.

Self-doubt sets in

But chronic obstructive pulmonary disease, or COPD, is a disease that I barely understood. Gradually, the acronym became more familiar and it began to dawn on me that I was not alone in the universe. There were many other people with diagnosed or undiagnosed lung problems — — 35 to 40 million of them, actually, a group so large that it seemed like an underclass in American society. Eventually I would learn more about COPD from reading and by talking with home health care specialists and such luminaries as Denver pulmonary pioneer, the late Dr. Thomas Petty, and New York pulmonologist, author, and former head of the American Lung Association, Dr. Neil Schachter. Nevertheless, in 2004 I was a neophyte unfamiliar with COPD in its various forms and unfamiliar with the history of oxygen portability.

I began to feel doubt as the reality of the trip approached. I doubted my ability to speak coherently, not to mention eloquently, on behalf of others who suffered from COPD. Although I had always kept myself in good physical shape, I also questioned whether or not I had the physical strength it would take to ride across the continent. Would I have the willpower it took to overcome physical and emotional obstacles associated with the trip? Would I decide to quit on days when I "hit the wall" and thus disappoint everyone involved? Looking back on it now, I can understand that the worries were just stage fright.

But there wasn't much time to worry. The cross-country bicycle trip would begin in San Francisco's Lincoln Park during the second week in July 2004. Ardath would drive the support vehicle and she and I would traverse the country together keeping notes and logs and taking photographs as we chipped away the miles. We drove our van to San Francisco where, prior to the sendoff, I performed the obligatory cross-country bicycling rituals: dipping the rear tire of my bike in the ocean and scooping up seawater in a small medicine bottle that we would carry across the country and empty into the Atlantic.

On a Saturday morning in July, a small group of well-wishers gathered on a sidewalk in Lincoln Park. Among them were Tyco and Mallinckrodt representatives, Nellcor Puritan-Bennett President Randy Whitfield, a representative of the American Lung Association, and a representative of ThirdAge, an organization that promotes the well being and self-development of middle-age people who are not quite ready to call themselves seniors. Following speeches from members of the respiratory health chorus, I got up to speak. With a lump in my throat, I explained how I had arrived at this point. Then came a pause. I wanted to express my gratitude to everyone but choked up. The words would not come out. After an embarrassing interlude, I expressed my thanks to the ineffable powers that be for giving me an opportunity to help others.

Fifteen Puritan-Bennett employees wearing "Helios Freedom Tour" biking shirts straddled their bikes, waiting patiently. The group, which included 13-year-old Michael Benko, whose ride would earn him a Boy Scout merit badge, would ride with me during the first day of the Freedom Tour. Radiating warmth, these fellow bicyclists seemed pleased and intrigued by the Tour. I knew that without the portable oxygen

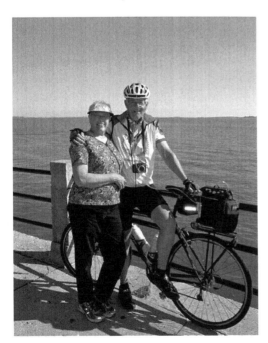
Mark & Ardath

system that they manufactured, my cross- country dream was a nonsensical whim. Even though we barely had time to become acquainted, I felt a bond drawing me to these people who earn their daily bread producing devices that improve the lives of oxygen-dependent people.

After leading our bicycling troupe in a circle around the parking lot fountain a couple of times for the benefit of media photographers, I headed downhill toward San Francisco Bay on my touring bicycle. Attached to a rack over the rear tire was my lightweight, Helios liquid oxygen canister turned up to its highest rate of 4 lpm. The once-personal odyssey, now a corporate-sponsored coast-to-coast Helios Freedom Tour, was underway. I would try to demonstrate how the use of supplemental oxygen leads to greater human productivity for the benefit of society.

The details of the trip are extensive. However, they can be read in a forthcoming book. In this chapter I will offer only a brief trip overview that may be relevant to fellow oxyphiles.

The tough spots

Bill Roe, a Davis, California realtor who rode his bicycle along the same Lincoln Highway route and detailed the trip in his book, All the Way to Lincolnway (Bill Roe, 2000) told me that my first major obstacle would be the Sierra Nevada mountain range. If I could surmount that obstacle, I ought to be confident about riding clear across the country. Bill was right. With Ardath driving our Volkswagen Eurovan and attending to every trip detail except pedaling the bicycle, I gained confidence each day following our departure from the Bay Area.

Beyond Sacramento, the route up into the foothills of the Sierra Nevada was a forest road flanking Interstate 80. The two-lane, asphalt path snaked upward through the pines, following the cataracts of a mountain stream, along a steeper grade than the interstate. At one point, inhaling rapidly through my oxygen cannula at the maximum rate of 4 lpm, I had to stop on a steep climb because my legs and lungs were not equal to the task. The steep climb required many pauses to allow me to catch my breath. Eventually, where the road petered out I had no option except to venture onto Interstate 80. I joined the Reno-Sacramento traffic, pedaling along the interstate shoulder for 17 miles on a gentler, steadier climb.

As I ascended toward the 7,085-foot Donner Summit of the Sierra Nevada Range I experienced a drop in oxygen saturation to just 84, but it was not worrisome. Because I had been living in a city situated at 6,100 feet above sea level, I expected my oxygen level to drop and I knew the feeling when it happened — an ache that bisected the top of my skull. The solution to the problem was to take a break when the grade became too strenuous and my lungs could not keep up with the effort. Gradually, after frequent stops, I reached the summit and coasted downhill rapidly toward an aqua jewel named Donner Lake. I had overcome the first obstacle in my quest.

More mountains, then the flat Midwest

Following the Sierra Nevadas, the major hurdles in the western portion of the Freedom Tour were the parallel set of mountain ranges across the width of Nevada, the Bonneville Salt Flats and Wasatch Range in Utah, and a 400 mile-long traverse of my home state of Wyoming along a route that averages approximately 7,000 feet above sea level. Together, they are major Western geographic landmarks not only for bicyclists, but also for travelers in steel-encased vehicles.

I navigated this route with few problems at a 4 lpm flow and keeping my sats in the 87-90 range.

East from Cheyenne, Wyoming, the altitude drops gradually in Nebraska to the point where, eventually, the only hills worth mention are the on-ramps to bridges over highways, railroads, or rivers. The Midwest states are generally flat or rolling and Illinois and Indiana, whose landscapes were scoured by glaciers, seemed the flattest. For an oxygen-dependent person, the topographic change from Western mountains and prairies to the Great Plains and Mississippi River bottomland means more oxygen and, thus, easier riding if one excludes the problem of occasional narrow road shoulders. At this point in the journey, I kept my liter flow at the maximum of 4 lpm but my oxygen saturation rose to above 90.

Bill Roe had warned me about the Alleghenies. Although the entire Appalachian chain is older and more eroded than the Rockies, the climb would not be easy. He was right. In eastern Ohio and western Pennsylvania one long climb followed another, requiring a flow of 4 lpm. Even though the altitudes of the summits are negligible, they are still long grinds for bicyclists. It was not until coasting down the east side of the Alleghenies toward the coastal tidewater region of the country that I became assured that the rest of the Lincoln Highway route would be flat.

The end run

From Philadelphia east the Lincoln Highway crosses the Delaware River and slices through the New Jersey landscape. The 2004 Helios Freedom Tour came to an end at Statue of Liberty Park on the Jersey side of New York Harbor.

Standing on rock riprap, I dipped my front tire in the cold water of the Atlantic Ocean and poured Pacific seawater from the bottle we had carried across the country. I had just completed a transcontinental bicycle ride. I felt a sense of accomplishment but a feeling of elation escaped me. Rather, my feeling was one of dull numbness. It would take at least another day that included a ferry ride to Manhattan and a short bicycle ride into Times Square, before I felt real joy in the accomplishment.

The following day, at a Tyco-sponsored celebration near Times Square, speeches were made and checks were presented. On behalf of the trip, Tyco donated $10,000 to the American Lung Association and the same amount to my favorite charity, the Cheyenne Family YMCA. The significance of the transcontinental trip was beginning to soak into my consciousness.

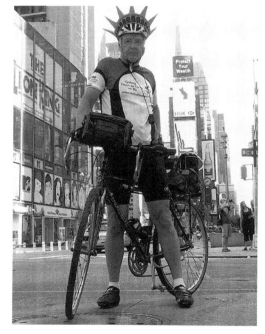

My life, reclaimed

The entire trip from San Francisco to New York was 3,400 miles and had taken nearly four months. The man riding his bike while inhaling supplemen-

Mark in New York City

tal oxygen had completed his self-appointed task and he may have been the first oxygen-dependent person to cross the country on a bicycle. However, that fact is irrelevant in the wide view of life. The Guinness Book of World Records is full of accomplishments irrelevant to our daily lives.

Besides, mine was not the accomplishment of a single individual or a feat comparable to the saga of Odysseus. Twenty-first century America is a cornucopia of wealth and human kindness. Food, supplies, shelter, and goodwill are plentiful throughout the country. No, my trip was more like Andy Warhol's "15 minutes of fame."

After seven years of living on supplemental oxygen, I can now look back over that early period of my disability and understand it more easily. While I both fought and tried to ignore the COPD classification, I also had taken the opportunity to reclaim my life. It took a while but my attitude changed. Blood clots were only a dent in the structure of life, just another turn in life's circuitous road. An inner voice advised: "Here's another opportunity. Try not to blow it."

Each morning when I return home after a short walk to the newspaper box, I look toward the east at the rising sun, thanking the ineffable powers that be. I thank them for granting me one more day and ask for the strength to help others. I continue to feel strongly that oxygen-dependent people should be encouraged to fulfill their lives, and I hope that I have done something to inspire them to achieve their own dreams.

"*You do not cease to fish because you get old,*
You get old because you cease to fish!"
— unknown —

Chapter 11

Flying the Friendly Skies
to Eastern Europe

Vlady Rozenbaum, PhD

Travel has always been one of my passions. Despite suffering from lung disease since I was a small child in Poland, I never felt limited in any way to pursue travel.

This changed in the mid 1990s when my wife and I visited the very pleasant Cote d'Azur resort of Menton in France. At that time, I was not yet on oxygen. During our vacation I noticed that I was getting tired more quickly than usual and I began trying to avoid longer walks.

On our flight back home to the U.S., I experienced some tightness in my chest that later changed into mild pain. I asked a flight attendant about the availability of a physician onboard. Well, there were four of them, all eager to help. One of them, an emergency physician, took charge. After a brief examination he gave me a pill and assured me that I was in no danger. I went back to my seat and the pain in my chest subsided. I left the plane feeling rather shaky, but luckily did not have a medical emergency on my flight from France.

Oxygen, 15 hours a day

It took another ten years before I was ready to fly overseas again. By then I knew that I must not fly without oxygen, even on domestic flights. I also realized that I should discuss my travel by air with a doctor.

According to a recent study, 18% of passengers with COPD experience at least mild respiratory distress during a flight.[1] Even passengers with mild COPD find their oxygenation noticeably reduced. Therefore, it is generally recommended that people with a resting oxygen saturation of 92-95%

arrange for in-flight oxygen supplementation.[2]

I have very severe COPD (FEV$_1$ at 26%) and I use oxygen more than 15 hours a day. At night the oxygen line is attached to my CPAP machine as I suffer from obstructive sleep apnea as well. At rest I use oxygen on and off from a stationary oxygen concentrator (continuous flow) at 1-2 lpm.

I check my saturation occasionally with a Nonin finger oximeter to make sure that I get enough oxygen. My night liter flow is at 3 lpm.

For activity I use a light portable oxygen unit providing a pulse mode. Usually, setting 2 is sufficient, but sometimes I go to 3. I have been using supplementary oxygen for some 15 years now (the first few years only at night) and I can easily determine by my breathing when I need to increase the setting. I make sure to verify it with an oximeter.

It is very important to remember that mastering breathing techniques (diaphragmatic, pursed-lip, and slowing down the breathing rate) make the use of portable oxygen equipment much more effective. It is recommended to use a higher liter flow in the air than on the ground. With portable oxygen concentrators (POCs) this may be somewhat problematic as their settings sometimes DO NOT correspond to liter flow. I have not experienced any problems with my oxygen level in the air when using settings 2 or 3. However, this may not be sufficient for others with very advanced lung disease.

Perhaps I should mention here that there are pre-flight assessment tests available in some clinics. One is called the hypoxic inhalation test, or HIT. Sometimes a 50-meter walk is used for this purpose as well.[3] However, I have never had a pre-flight assessment test.

Off to Poland

In 2006, Professor Jan Zielinski, an eminent Polish pulmonologist and a member of COPD-ALERT, mentioned the upcoming annual conference of the Polish Society of Pulmonologists in an email to me. The program was very interesting and I was additionally intrigued by the location of the conference. It was to take place in Opole, a historic city in southwestern Poland known for annual song festivals.

My wife, who likes to travel with me to conferences and is always of great help, decided to check with the Polish LOT Airlines about their policy for passengers requiring in-flight oxygen. We were elated to find out that LOT Airlines offered free oxygen. The procedure was simple. One just needed to download the Medical Information Sheet (MEDIF) from the LOT Airlines website and submit it to his/her physician for completion.

The form contained questions about the passenger's medical condition and need for medical devices and oxygen. (Liter flow and the duration of use had to be specified.) Upon completion of the form, the doctor was required to affix his/her stamp and signature at the bottom, and then fax it to the LOT Airlines office. The stamp was very important; my doctor's first form was rejected because his stamp was missing.

Then came the tricky part. The form was only valid for two weeks, which would not cover my entire trip! What can you do if you have a chronic lung condition and do not know any doctor in Poland? After arguing for a little while with the LOT Airlines staff that my chronic condition is permanent, I was told that the two-week validity requirement may not be strictly enforced in Warsaw. However, just in case, I took a couple of blank MEDIF forms with me.

POCs make it easy

Since we live in the Washington, DC, area, we decided to take a train to Newark, NJ, where we could take a direct LOT Airlines flight to Warsaw. The cost of the oxygen equipment that we would need to rent in Poland was too high (and the equipment we wanted was not readily available). Because of this we took two portable oxygen concentrators (POCs) with us: the SeQual Eclipse (to be used as a stationary concentrator at night) and the AirSep FreeStyle (with a strap-on extra battery) for activity.

I was able to use FreeStyle in the car, on the train, at the train station, and at the airport. There was no problem finding an electric outlet to plug it into. Checking in at the airport went smoothly. Nobody made any comments about the FreeStyle, even at the security counter. Needless to say, I used a wheelchair at the airport. It really simplifies moving around and allows for much faster security check. Always request the wheelchair at the time of ticketing.

Boarding the plane was not a problem, but once we were seated, we did experience one little glitch. The crew knew that I would be using oxygen, but they were not in a hurry to give it to me. I had to remind them several times after we took off. Apparently, they thought that I would need oxygen only for some portions of the flight. After we clarified the misunderstanding, I received an oxygen cylinder with a shoulder strap and a face mask with a hose. The cylinder was made in the United States by Avox Systems, which specializes in medical oxygen support for the aviation industry.

Small cylinders make a difference

A flight attendant connected the hose and opened the valve. I replaced the face mask with my own nasal cannula for greater comfort. The entire flight required 4-5 cylinders (they had to be changed every two hours). These smaller cylinders were very convenient as they allowed me to move around the plane without any problem.

It made me wonder why we could not be provided with such cylinders on our domestic flights. At the time — before POCs were approved for use on commercial airlines — we would instead be given big cylinders, which were placed in the overhead compartment or under the seat. When we had

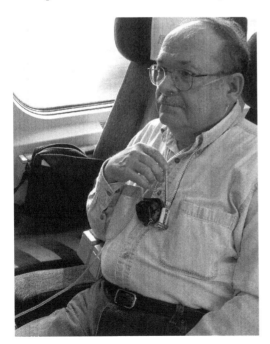

to go to the restroom, we had to remove the cannula, which resulted in quick desaturation. Sometimes my oxygenation would have dropped to as low as 74% saturation by the time I got back to my seat. I know this because I was using my personal oximeter.

We landed safely in Poland, and my oxygen equipment arrived in perfect condition as well. I was happy to see that both Eclipse and FreeStyle automatically converted to the different voltage in the Warsaw apartment where we were staying. Moving around in Warsaw was quite easy

Train travel

because of a very good public transportation system. Occasionally we had to use taxicabs, and if the cab driver found the POC and clicking noises suspicious, I only had to explain what was going on and the driver was always very understanding.

On the street, in shopping malls and restaurants, and on public transportation, the POC sounds blended smoothly with the urban noises. Nobody was bothered by my POC and I did not get funny looks. The FreeStyle output was, for the most part, sufficient, although during some challenging walks (stairs, uneven pavement, etc.) my oxygenation was barely at 90%.

Too many stairs

Accommodations for the handicapped are not always available in Poland, so I had plenty of opportunity to use effective breathing techniques. To get to Opole for the pulmonology conference we decided to take a fast train from Warsaw. I was able to plug in my FreeStyle. The trouble started when we arrived in Opole late in the evening. There were no elevators or escalators to take us from the platform to the railroad station's main hall. We had to use stairs three times to get onto the street. There was nobody to help us with our luggage. When we managed to reach the street there were no cabs waiting, and by that time there was no public transportation available. It took a good while before a cab driver decided to try his luck and see if there were any passengers who may need a ride.

The conference was well organized. No more issues with transportation. A special shuttle bus took us from the hotel to the meetings. There were many interesting panels, and in the evenings we enjoyed concerts by top Polish entertainers. However, we were quite shocked to see many smoking pulmonologists. Apparently, this is a serious problem among Polish medical professionals and special smoking cessation counseling was offered at the conference to help them quit.

Lessons learned

On our way back to Warsaw we were smarter. Instead of pulling the Eclipse in a suitcase (to protect it from the elements), we removed it so I could use it while "negotiating" the stairs at the train station. That worked great. Eclipse's bigger oxygen bolus made it easier for me to walk the stairs. Then in the middle of our climb we were offered assistance by a man walking behind us. It turned out that he was also returning to Warsaw from the same conference. He recognized my equipment and we had a nice conversation about oxygen therapy.

His name was Jan Kus and he happened to be the chief of the First Clinical Department at the very prestigious Institute of Tuberculosis and Lung Diseases in Warsaw. Professor Kus invited me to give a presentation to his medical staff. I was very flattered and excited. It was there, in 1952, that I had had a successful surgery for bronchiectasis. I spent a month in the hospital and a year recuperating from the surgery.

For the presentation I decided to wear the Oxy-View glasses that make the use of oxygen more discreet. *(See Presentation photo)* It worked! When Professor Kus told the assembled physicians that I was on oxygen and asked them to guess how it was delivered, they could not tell.

Heading home, and back again

Our stay in Poland was enjoyable. We had a chance to visit with my in-laws and with old friends. Before we left we had to confirm our reservations and oxygen arrangements. That took two days, because of the discussion of the validity of the MEDIF form (the two week expiration date, remember?) and computer glitches (LOT Airlines is hooked up to three computer networks that do not communicate very well with each other).

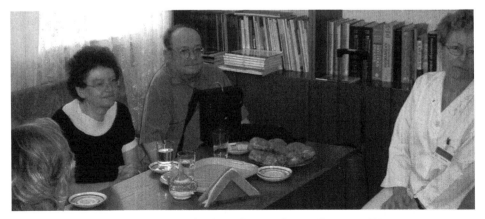

Staff presentation at the Institute of Tuberculosis and Lung Diseases, Warsaw.

Still, when I boarded the plane there was no oxygen for me. A flight attendant looking at my FreeStyle asked me: "What's the problem? You have your own oxygen!" I told him that my batteries would not last long enough and handed him a newly completed MEDIF form with a signature and the stamp of a professor of respiratory diseases (which I had arranged for in advance, just in case). That worked like a charm and I got my oxygen.

These minor problems with the LOT Airlines did not discourage me from future visits. Shortly after my return I was invited by the Polish Academy of Sciences to participate in an international conference on the Sovietization of Eastern Europe after World War II. Needless to say, I did not hesitate to accept it. The location was great: Szklarska Poreba, a spa in the mountains of southern Poland where I had vacationed as a teenager 50 years earlier. This invitation also allowed me to put on my other hat, that of a historian.

Another great trip

Again I took the Eclipse and FreeStyle concentrators with me. I decided to take both of them on board this time, but I was using free oxygen furnished by LOT Airlines. The Eclipse fit very easily under the seat in front of me. As usual, there were no electrical outlets at our seats to try the POCs. A friendly flight attendant was curious to find out how they worked and offered me her seat with an electrical outlet so we could test the equipment. Both POCs performed well. To show my gratitude I checked her oxygenation with my Nonin. It showed 93%! The lady became somewhat alarmed and asked what she could do about it. "Quit smoking!" suggested a male flight attendant standing with us. I recommended that she visit a pulmonologist. (Editorial note: Saturation of 93% is considered within normal range in Denver, Colorado, at an altitude of 5,280 ft.

Upon arrival in Warsaw we did not realize that the plane did not dock with the hub and we had to walk down the steps to reach the ground. If we had known that, I would have requested a wheelchair. The experience was physically taxing, and being attached to the Eclipse, which I had to drag along with the FreeStyle on my shoulder, did not help much. I was very short of breath by the time I reached the ground. It is always important to ask about services at the airport when making your flight arrangements.

We again visited with family in Warsaw (this time only my mother in-law was still alive) and with friends. To get to Szklarska Poreba we took a fast train to Wroclaw and from there a charter bus took us to the conference site. The conference was very interesting, even though no entertainment was offered. The weather was terrible, however — pouring rain almost the entire time, so I could not revisit some old places.

Polish-U.S. symposium

During my visit the year before I noticed that the pulmonology conference had been preceded by a Polish-Ukrainian symposium. I suggested a Polish-U.S. conference on COPD. Professor Zielinski liked the idea and asked me to help entice several eminent U.S. pulmonologists to attend.

It turned out that my job was not difficult at all. At the invitation of the Polish Academy of Sciences and the Warsaw Medical University, Drs. Richard Casaburi, Bartolome Celli, and Richard ZuWallack joined me in presenting papers at the Polish-U.S. symposium on reducing the burden of COPD in October of 2008. In the evening the U.S. participants were given a splendid tour of Warsaw's Old City in horse-drawn carts and treated to a lavish dinner at a famous restaurant.

The next day my wife and I were hosted by Professor Ewa Nizankowska-Mogilnicka, chief of the pulmonary clinic at the Jagiellonian University Medical School in Krakow, in southern Poland. Two doctors took us on walking tours of the surrounding area (the historic Jewish Quarter) and the clinic.

BYOE (Bring your own equipment)

When traveling to Eastern Europe one has to keep in mind less frequent accommodations for people with disabilities and steep prices for oxygen equipment and deliveries. That's why it is wise to bring your own equipment. Furthermore, as of the end of 2008, LOT Airlines stopped offering free oxygen. One has to buy it from the airline. This decision could have been precipitated by the aforementioned U.S. Department of Transportation regulation (Title 14 CFR Part 382) which, as of May 13, 2009, obligates all airlines domestic and foreign (if their flights originate or end in the United States) to permit passengers to use their own POCs so long as they are approved by the Federal Aviation Administration.

I would encourage fellow travelers to research the availability of oxygen for air travel as well as international airline regulations before embarking on an overseas trip. A very interesting recent study out of New Zealand looked at current regulations on in-flight supplemental oxygen for passengers with lung diseases. The authors examined 54 commercial airlines servicing international routes. Some of these airlines have flights into and out of the United States. The study focused on oxygen delivery, approvals required, equipment, and cost.[4]

Closer to home

The Polish-U.S. conference on COPD marked my last trip to Eastern Europe. There were too many travels to undertake here at home. I must say that, in my experience, traveling with a companion makes a lot of difference. My wife accompanies me on all trips, and her assistance and support make them much more enjoyable.

References

1. Coker RK, Shiner RJ, Partridge MR. "Is air travel safe for those with lung disease?" Eur Respir J 2007;30:1057-63.

2. Silverman D, Gendreau M. "Medical issues associated with commercial flights." Lancet 2009; 373:2067-2077.

3. Darwish AAM. Aerospace Medicine: Part 4. The Internet Journal of Pulmonary Medicine 2003;3(2).

4. Walker J, Kelly PT, Beckert L. "Airline policy for passengers requiring supplemental in-flight oxygen." Respirology 2009;14(4):589-594.

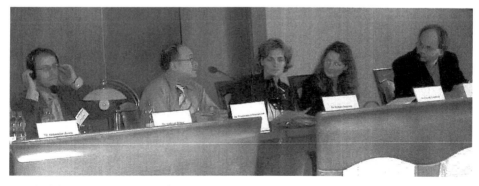

Panel of the International Conference on Cold War in Eastern Europe

"Even if you've been fishing for three hours and haven't gotten anything except poison ivy and sunburn, you're still better off than the worm."

— unknown —

Chapter 12

Patient Support Groups
and Activities

Mary R. Burns, R.N., B.S.

There are advantages to growing older. Perhaps the best is being able to look back over the years and see that the long hours, hard work and frustrations of dealing with bureaucrats were all worth the effort.

I am a fervent supporter and advocate of pulmonary rehabilitation programs. An enthusiastic staff, supportive pulmonary physician and cooperative hospital administration are key elements in the success of such a program. But in patient support groups the patient is often the key element in the group's success. It is almost with a sense of awe that I realize what has been accomplished over the years with the enthusiastic support and encouragement of my wonderful patients. Never underestimate the power of the patient!

Can you imagine being enthusiastic and ready to participate in group projects when even getting out of the house may be a struggle? Let's be realistic and admit that most people with significant respiratory disease understandably are discouraged, depressed and short of breath with even minimal activity. We can live for weeks with limited amounts of food, days with limited water, but only a very few minutes without air. Shortness of breath is not easy to ignore.

That is why pulmonary rehabilitation is so important for those fortunate enough to live in an area that offers it. Even the most debilitated patients can be greatly helped.

We now know that COPD is a multi organ disease, which affects the muscles long before shortness of breath becomes noticeable. Everyone needs to exercise but it is as essential as medication for those with COPD. While repairing damage to the lungs may not be possible, getting muscles back in shape is very doable. It's hard for anyone to start an exercise program. Who would even consider it when they also are short of breath? Not many. That is where a pulmonary rehabilitation program can benefit patients.

The first order of business is learning how to control shortness of breath and prevent panic attacks that understandably discourage exercise. Breathing retraining starts the first day of class, or even during the initial interview, and continues until the last day. Exercise reconditioning starts slowly. It may start with walking a few minutes 5 times a day while practicing good breathing techniques and pacing. Strengthening exercises are gradually added along with energy conservation and educational classes on everything from medications to travel. Exercise duration and strength rapidly increase as tolerated. The tremendous improvement in body and spirit that can be accomplished after just a few weeks in pulmonary rehabilitation is mind-boggling.

The other big benefit of a pulmonary rehab program is the friendships that can develop with others in a class. Many continue to communicate and support each other after the program is completed. This is made even easier when the rehab program has an established support group to join. If there isn't one, perhaps you might consider now is the time for organizing one of your own.

While organizational assistance from a hospital and health care professionals is very helpful, small, autonomous patient groups can also accomplish a great deal. I will relate some of the things the PEP Pioneers patient support group accomplished in the hope that this will give you some ideas for your group.

The PEP Pioneers

The first graduates of the Pulmonary Education Program (PEP) at Little Company of Mary Hospital in Torrance, California formed a support group. They called themselves the PEP Pioneers. Back in the mid 1970s these patients were truly pioneers. One of the founding members had started a local Alcoholics Anonymous (AA) group and brought to the Pioneers much of the AA philosophy of helping each other. It was an inspired idea. They reached out to even the most grumpy, depressed, and needy newcomer. Everyone was welcome and blossomed in this nourishing atmosphere.

A telephone committee was formed to keep in regular touch with all members. Monthly support group meetings were held, at first in a local restaurant. As the group expanded, meetings moved to a room in the hospital; speakers were invited, often with personal physicians as guest lecturers. Birthdays and holidays were celebrated with special decorations. New graduates of the rehab program were honored guests and officially made Pioneers. White elephants, home baked goods, fruits and vegetables from gardens were used as prizes for the monthly raffle, proceeds going to the club. The non-pulmonary spouse or significant other was not only included but was a tremendous help and important contributor to the success of the group.

In those days there was no place to exercise after rehab was completed, so it was important to find ways to facilitate regular exercise. Local parks and malls were carefully measured and drawn with distances, rest stops, and those important bathrooms identified. The maps were printed, distributed, and a group formed to walk together. Special encouragement and support were always given to the patient newly on oxygen, often uncomfortable with being seen in public back in the days when it was still rare to see someone using oxygen.

Finding good places to walk indoors in inclement weather was a problem. Local malls seemed ideal, though it took some time to convince mall managers of that! Finally in 1981 the first of two large malls established early hours, just for our patients, with distances marked every 10 feet on the walking areas. Patients were able to keep track of distances walked, turning in the total at monthly meetings for acknowledgement and token prizes. A politician and minor TV star celebrated the grand opening of the indoor walking area with a ribbon cutting ceremony. Good publicity made this more attractive to reluctant mall managers as well as to our ribbon cutters. Patients were on a roll. This was the first mall in the world to have a measured walking area for pulmonary patients.

The more patients became involved, the more enthusiastic they became and the better they felt. An annual potluck picnic was started. Bus trips to local attractions were organized for the group. Many of them had been home bound before starting pulmonary rehabilitation, afraid of running out of oxygen. Stationary systems and extra portable units were brought along, furnished by a local Durable Medical Equipment (DME) company, so being on oxygen no longer meant being stuck within a four hour radius of home.

The Respiratory Rally

Despite these accomplishments, the President of the support group sorrowfully asked, "Are we out here all alone?" This inspired the idea for the first Respiratory Rally back in 1981. Patients, families and health care professionals from all over Southern California were invited to join us for a day of fun, education, and fellowship. Education was important, but sharing an enjoyable day was the real goal.

The original grandiose idea was to have a Respiratory Olympics. Among other events, we settled for a more realistic Pace Race. The object was to guess how long it would take to complete a short measured walk without getting short of breath. The most debilitated patient on oxygen could, and usually did, win. They had learned to pace themselves during rehab. Doctors are sadly lacking in this skill. They usually came in last, much to the delight of their patients.

One of our patients made Dr. Tom Petty an honorary PEP Pioneer and begged him to attend a Rally so many times he finally agreed. The energy and happiness of so many people on oxygen delighted him as it had other pulmonary physicians, who so often see only those who are sick and depressed. Dr. Petty became a regular, beloved guest speaker at all Rallies in the years that followed.

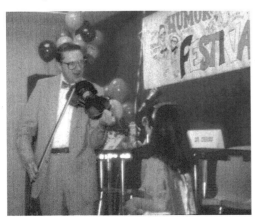

Respiratory Rally

Each Rally had a different theme ranging from *Pioneer Days* to the very popular *Humor for the Health of It*. Education was important but guest speakers were required to include a minimum of three jokes in every talk given at a Rally. Their attempts to include a joke were sometimes funnier than the jokes themselves and the audience loved it. Dr. Petty, of course, had a never-ending repertoire for his appreciative audience. These Rallies became an annual event that growing numbers of support groups looked forward to, reserving buses so their entire group could travel together. Oxygen companies refilled and topped off portable units for the ride home. Local stores and restaurants donated gifts that could be raffled off. Hospital volunteers blew up balloons, passed out lunches, or even dressed as clowns greeting guests arriving by car and bus. Local respiratory therapy and nursing students were eager volunteers helping with an attendance that increased to over three hundred participants most years. "*What a fun day!*" and "*See you next year!*" are what we heard again and again as smiling, laughing guests departed.

Cruising With Oxygen

Did you know that back in 1984 medical oxygen was considered hazardous cargo, and not allowed on cruise ships? We didn't, so when one of my patients begged me to arrange a cruise I innocently answered, "Sure." I now understand the aphorism, which says fools rush in where angels fear to tread. If I had the faintest idea of what I was getting into, that cruise never would have happened. But I didn't know and naively continued to plan this first cruise for oxygen patients. Three weeks before sailing, when we rechecked with the cruise line, we found to our horror that the tourist agency had told them nothing about our plans to take oxygen on board.

Oxygen use was illegal for even a visitor on a cruise line. The cruise was off. Our tourist agents, eager for the commissions from our group of 52, encouraged us to "sneak on board," or "run past the ticket taker at the last minute." A vision of our patients running up gangways pulling their oxygen, pursued by ticket agents, was not what we had in mind for this dream trip!

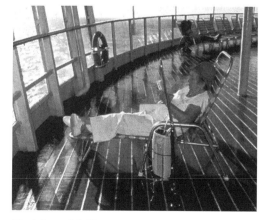

Cruising with Oxygen

After inundating them with safety information, *and* a powerful letter from Dr. Petty darkly hinting at the perils of discrimination, we finally convinced the reluctant SS Azure Seas to allow us on board with oxygen, IF we could get Coast Guard approval. Everyone was positive we would never budge that bureaucracy or change the law. But, miracles really do happen, especially when you work very hard to achieve them. In a frantic three-week period, all obstacles were overcome. The local Coast Guard approved the trip. On June 11, 1984, we sailed from San Pedro, CA to Ensenada, Mexico. For the first time in history, passengers with oxygen were allowed on a cruise ship. Oxygen dependent passengers have been cruising the world ever since.

Wonderful things began to happen in that ocean air. Patients who had hated upper extremity exercises in rehab would play the one armed bandits by the hour, with nary a complaint. Those who "couldn't" handle stairs managed very nicely, with their portable oxygen, to climb the half flight up to the casino.

Many amusing incidents happened on this first trip. Other passengers thought our patients with portable oxygen units were using miniature vacuum cleaners on *"the cleanest ship ever seen."* A hissing oxygen tank convinced one panicked steward we were about to blow up the ship. Waiters carefully extinguished our flaming Baked Alaska before serving it to our group on the last night of the cruise. We gave them an extra tip for volunteering for the "hazardous duty" of serving our group on oxygen.

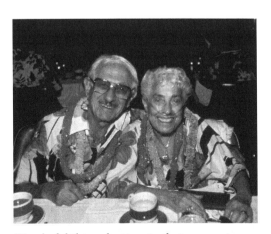

Wonderful things happen in that ocean air.

How times and attitudes have change! What *hasn't* changed is the fun people have when cruising. Some of our group found that oxygen was no deterrent to swimming when using extension tubing, and learned to again enjoy the pool. Another couple danced on deck, thanks to extension tubing on the oxygen tank, while onlookers burst into appreciative applause.

Our entire group attended the Captain's Dinner Dance. They proudly posed with their oxygen, resplendent in their evening clothes, for the inevitable picture by the boat photographer. Who said being on oxygen was the end of a fun life? They didn't! They danced, carrying their own oxygen or having their partner carry it. It didn't matter; they were having fun. So, the next time those of you on oxygen go on a cruise, remember the struggles it took to legalize this, way back in the dark ages of 1984, and enjoy!

Our patients came back from that cruise bursting with energy and planning their next cruise. The exhausted pulmonary staff went home and collapsed, not yet realizing what we had accomplished.

Of the fifty-two travelers on our first cruise, twenty-four were on oxygen and almost all had serious lung damage. The word began to spread in the pulmonary community about what had been accomplished. A call came from a rehabilitation program in Kansas City, MO. They urged us to arrange a joint Caribbean cruise with them, meeting in Miami. Pushed by enthusiastic patients, we agreed. We needed to fly our patients, many on oxygen, from Los Angeles to Miami and back again to accomplish this. Again things went relatively well until the last two weeks. Disaster struck again. Both the airlines and the cruise line decided it was too dangerous and cancelled our reservations. Once again, with the help of Dr. Petty and many others who intervened, they reluctantly were convinced to give us a try. The 1985 cruise was on and again a huge success. Our well-screened and supervised patients did much better than usual passengers the ships allowed. The cruise lines were now convinced oxygen patients could safely be allowed and happily anticipated a surge in passengers on oxygen

The National Coast Guard in Washington, DC, fortunately ignorant of our two previous cruises, belatedly learned of them by reading an article I wrote in the Journal of Nursing. They were rather upset. An edict was issued. Passengers with oxygen were flatly forbidden on all ships. After months of being bombarded with additional documentation and testimonials, they finally relented. Oxygen use by passengers on ships was henceforth legal.

Dr. Petty invited me to speak about these cruises in Denver to an international audience of almost one thousand physicians and healthcare professionals interested in pulmonary rehabilitation. My feet were so slick with nervous perspiration that I skidded across the floor to the mike. To my huge relief, everyone was as excited about our cruises as I was. Even better, they were additionally interested in our use of portable oxygen and the pulmonary rehabilitation that had improved severely impaired patients enough to enjoy such a trip. It triggered the start of a stream of visitors to our facility from around the world. Letters and requests to speak on rehabilitation and oxygen, as well as cruises and travel, began arriving. Our cruise had ignited a firestorm of interest in pulmonary rehabilitation and portable oxygen as well as travel.

One of our first visitors was Dr. Jan Zelinski of Poland *(see Chapter 16)* who spoke to our fascinated patient support group. He returned to Warsaw to start the first pulmonary rehabilitation program behind the Iron Curtain and proudly arranged a day-long boat ride on the Vistula River. He had no funds, so for years we sent him our outdated but still good equipment, including an oximeter, possibly the first behind the Iron Curtain. It enabled him to do some wonderful research. He dedicated some of his research publications to our PEP Pioneers. He is still a good friend.

Dr. Freddy Smeets visited us several times from Belgium, also interested by the Denver presentation. It took only one afternoon at the PEP patient club, listening to enthusiastic patients on oxygen, to make him a believer. He also went home to start annual cruises, but outdid us by holding his Respiratory Rally in a local castle!

Many more guests visited us to observe for themselves if our oxygen patients were really as active as I claimed in the lectures now being given at international symposiums. They were often so impressed with our active patient group that they returned again or invited me to their countries to speak. Physicians came from areas as far apart as Tromso, Norway, 600 miles above the Arctic Circle, Japan and New Zealand on the other side of the world. We all had a great deal in common. We wanted to improve the lives of patients with COPD and help those on oxygen live better lives.

PERF, The Pulmonary Education and Research Foundation

A very special patient in those early days was Mary Grancell. Mary, like all of those first Pioneers, became a close friend. She was very important in developing the group, supporting me, and a wonderful example of what someone can achieve even when on oxygen. After her death, her husband

Alvin wished to further pulmonary rehabilitation and to help improve lives of other pulmonary patients the way hers had been helped. That was the start of PERF, the Pulmonary Education and Research Foundation. The goal of PERF is to focus on practical projects and research, and to bring benefits to pulmonary patients in the short term. Led by Presidents, such as Dr. Thomas Petty and Dr. Richard Casaburi, this small foundation succeeded in that goal with some amazing achievements.

PERF, thanks to Alvin Grancell, funded the Alvin Grancell-Mary Burns Chair in the Rehabilitative Sciences at the Los Angeles Biomedical Research Institute at Harbor-UCLA Medical Center in Torrance, California in 2000. This was the first Chair in the world dedicated to the study of pulmonary rehabilitation and needs of pulmonary patients. The Chair was permanently endowed in order to allow its occupant to reduce his or her clinical responsibilities. This would allow more time for research and spreading information about the value of pulmonary rehabilitation. As the first occupant of that Chair, Richard Casaburi, PhD, MD, has more than succeeded in that mission.

Another fund, established in 2008, is devoted to providing financial assistance for visiting scientists who come from countries around the world. They learn about pulmonary rehabilitation, oxygen and exercise while participating in research aimed at better understanding and helping those with pulmonary disease when they return to their country. Patients volunteer for these clinical trials considering them a win-win situation. Study participants are helped as much as the scientists working with them in the positive atmosphere of the Rehabilitation Clinical Trials Center.

I shouldn't quote a tobacco slogan but I can't resist. *We've come a long way, baby!* Clinical trials have proven the benefits of newer medications, along with pulmonary rehabilitation, exercise, oxygen, and support groups. Equally important, attitudes about the future of the pulmonary patient have become much more positive these past 25 years

The Future

So what is left to achieve? Unfortunately, a great deal. While pulmonary rehabilitation has spread around the world there are many places in the United States where good rehabilitation, and good support groups are not available. I hope that reading about what some pioneering patients accomplished thirty years ago will inspire you to start your own group, or to energize a support group you already have. The individual patient *can* make a difference!

What new ideas and opportunities do I see coming in the future? Why, taking advantage of, and making use of, all the technological advances that have exploded upon us in the past 10 years is sure to make a big difference. Friends in Norway, Sweden, Thailand and Japan all stay connected. Wouldn't it be interesting for your group to also contact those in other countries to see how they do rehabilitation or form support groups? The high standards and wonderful rehabilitation programs in some of these countries are so much like ours that you might be surprised.

As new patients with greater computer skills enter your support group the telephone committee may be improved or even replaced by Skype (a software application that allows users to make voice calls over the Internet). Patients with an exacerbation no longer need be isolated. Thanks to inexpensive computers and cameras, free group calls can be made and friends can be communicated with or even seen face to face when homebound.

How about keeping in touch with Facebook or one of the other social networks *(see Chapter 13)* A support group newsletter can be e-mailed monthly. Announcements can now be sent to everyone with the click of a key. Your group can develop its own web site to store names and contact information for group members. Lectures that are missed can be stored here. Your exercise diary can be recorded and reviewed on line. Classes can post lecture outlines and explanations. The possibilities are endless. Someone younger and more technologically advanced can probably think of many more exciting developments soon available.

Bad weather or distance need no longer separate us. Did you know some of the support groups in Japan would love to join some American support groups in Hawaii? Hawaiian groups are eager to host a Pan-Pacific Respiratory Rally. Support groups in California, Australia and Taiwan have already expressed interest in joining such an event. If that seems a little too ambitious, just meeting with groups in neighboring cities would be a great start.

The possibilities are endless. Let me end with a paraphrase from Dr. Petty.

"Remember to live and remember that you too can enjoy life with oxygen!"

Chapter 13

Adventures in COPD Advocacy and Awareness

Edna M. Fiore

My introduction to the respiratory world began in 1995 when I retired and moved from sea level in Newport, OR, to join my family in Conifer, CO, at an elevation of 8,500 feet. I had been spending vacations and holidays in Conifer for several years without any noticeable breathing problems, but within a short time I began to notice a little shortness of breath.

An advertisement in the Rocky Mountain News led me to Colorado Pulmonary Associates (CPA) and Dr. Tom Petty's research assistant, Wayne Silvers. A lifelong history of episodic asthma, a number of bouts with pneumonia, and a family history of respiratory problems combined with my status as a former smoker qualified me for a series of studies at CPA.

In 1998 I moved to Lakewood, a suburb of Denver, in order to be closer to the site of the research studies and resources for my own research as historian for the Town of Morrison and the Lariat Loop Heritage Alliance.

Medication makes a difference

Colorado proved to be the right place for someone with COPD. Historically, Colorado has been a national and world leader for the diagnosis and treatment of lung disease. From 1840 to 1920 it was considered the number one destination for people suffering from asthma and tuberculosis; as much as 60% of Colorado's early settlers migrated to the area seeking help for their respiratory ailments. National Jewish Health began serving respiratory patients in 1899 and has the distinction of being named the number one respiratory hospital by *U.S. News & World Report* for 11 consecutive years.

In 1999 I registered for research studies at National Jewish, where I was first introduced to tiotropium, a medication that I considered a "wonder drug." My stamina and endurance were easily doubled by it. My FEV_1 was hovering around 30% before I entered the study. At the conclusion of another tiotropium study in 2001 my FEV_1 had improved to 45%.

I continued to volunteer whenever and wherever a tiotropium study was offered. Fate smiled on me and I had the good fortune of receiving the study drug in all but one instance. By 2001 the wonder drug had acquired the trade name "Spiriva." In 2001 I participated in the pulmonary rehabilitation program at Exempla Lutheran in Wheat Ridge, CO, and was introduced to the world of collaborative self-management.

Oxygen enters the picture

I purchased a Nonin pulse oximeter in 2001 after learning about oxygen saturation levels in the pulmonary rehab program. But my personal odyssey with oxygen began in earnest in 2004 when I was prescribed O2 for sleep and exertion. In 2006 two exacerbations and a lung abscess drastically reduced my lung capacity, and although I still maintained an FEV1 of 40%, my daytime O2 saturation had slowly declined to just about 90%, so I was prescribed two liters of oxygen 24/7.

My oxygen set up consisted of an Invacare Platinum stationary concentrator and a liquid portable. The aftermath of the acute episodes had caused a paralysis of my diaphragm, with very shallow breathing, so I was unable to use the Helios, but found the Caire Spirit 300 suitable for my portable needs.

In October 2008 Inspired Technologies provided me with their new and innovative SmartDose portable, a Caire Spirit with the new SmartDose multi-valve feature that shapes the oxygen delivery to provide a gentle, quiet pulse when possible, but is also able to deliver a faster, high flow dose when needed. I have found that the SmartDose is ideal for my needs and allows me to live relatively carefree for everyday activities.

EFFORTS opens the door

I first discovered the larger COPD community back in 2002 when I was searching the Internet for a source in Europe where I could obtain

Spiriva. I clicked on www.emphysema.net and discovered the Emphysema Foundation For Our Right To Survive (EFFORTS) www.emphysema.net. EFFORTS opened a whole new world of information and support and started me on the path to COPD awareness and advocacy. I learned that EFFORTS held Rallies in Washington, DC, in 2000, 2001, and 2002, that brought COPD awareness to both legislative and public attention.

EFFORTS afforded me a "crash course" in COPD awareness, and within a very short time I was appointed EFFORTS state leader for Colorado. My first endeavor, with the help of Cindy Liverance, vice-president of the American Lung Association of Colorado, was an EFFORTS "Gathering" featuring a program about COPD research and general information at Lutheran Hospital in June of 2003.

The first U.S. COPD Coalition National Conference, already in the planning stages and set to be held in Arlington, VA, in conjunction with the second World COPD Day in November of 2003, was the next EFFORTS endeavor. I immediately made plans to attend! (EFFORTS President Linda Watson provides a detailed description of EFFORTS' activities at this event in Chapter 14.)

The encouragement and enthusiasm generated by this conference resulted in the first Colorado COPD Conference in 2004, which was planned by the Colorado COPD Network along with the National Emphysema/COPD Association. The theme was "COPD: Living the Colorado High Life." This conference has since become an annual event and in 2009 was officially designated the "Thomas L. Petty MD Moving Mountains COPD Conference."

Flying with O2

Another result of the U.S. COPD Coalition Conference and the EFFORTS Rallies was the formation of the Congressional COPD Caucus in 2004 by Senator Mike Crapo (ID). Representatives Cliff Stearns (FL) and John Lewis (GA), and Senator Blanche Lincoln (AR) joined Senator Crapo as caucus co-chairs.

The Congressional COPD Caucus gave the COPD community a public platform in Congress to bring attention to critical issues that have been identified by the U.S. COPD Coalition and the patient and professional COPD communities. The first issue addressed by the caucus was the difficulty of flying with supplementary oxygen. This resulted in the Federal Aviation Administration ruling on August 11, 2005, permitting the use of approved portable oxygen concentrators (POCs) on the airlines.

Frontier Airlines, with headquarters at Denver International Airport, was the first airline to permit POCs. Frontier produced a POC training film that featured Maryanne Hinderlide, a member of the original Colorado COPD Network, and her son, a Frontier flight attendant.

Change in prescription

The 6th Oxygen Consensus Conference in August of 2005 reached these conclusions: "Industry has continued to produce new ultra lightweight oxygen systems, which can truly be called 'ambulatory.' Low weight oxygen concentrators are making oxygen travel more practical and realistic for patients who require oxygen around the clock. At the very time that these advances are occurring, third party payers, mainly Medicare, are continuing to plan reductions in reimbursement for newer systems. A realistic reimbursement system is critical to the future of LTOT, which involves the lives of approximately 1.2 million Americans."

All along I had been, as Dr. Tom says, "titrating as I migrated" with my Nonin oximeter, and it was soon after the 6th Oxygen Consensus Conference that I noted that my 02 saturation was very gradually declining during exercise and that I required oxygen for longer and longer periods.

Red letter year

The year 2006 was a red letter year for COPD advocacy and awareness as Bartolome R. Celli, MD, presented his paper, "Chronic Obstructive Pulmonary Disease: From Unjustified Nihilism to Evidence-based Optimism," at the May American Thoracic Society (ATS) Conference. This landmark treatise worked wonders in removing the "blame the victim" smoking stigma and placing COPD, the fourth leading cause of death, on the same footing as other major health issues.

A second major factor that brought COPD awareness to national attention was the November launch by Boehringer Ingelheim of their television commercials for Spiriva, the first medication developed specifically for the treatment of COPD. These commercials depict the average COPD patient as vital, productive, and fully active, rather than the previously accepted stereotype of a wheezing oldster stumbling along with the aid of a walker.

Another milestone in 2006 was the creation of the Colorado COPD Coalition, which brought together a diverse group of stakeholders from all over the state, including health professionals, patients, research scientists, industry representatives, state officials, and caregivers. The coalition held a COPD Summit in May, and under the guidance of Keith Breese of the American Lung Association, prepared and began implementation of the Colorado State COPD Plan in 2006/2007.

The Colorado COPD Surveillance Report was developed and disseminated in 2007. Keith represented Colorado at the first State COPD Coalition and presented the Colorado State COPD Plan at the U.S. COPD Coalition meeting during the 2007 CHEST Conference. This plan has subsequently served as the prototype for the formation of many other state COPD coalitions.

High altitude adventure

On August 27, 2006, I had the privilege of joining 12 other intrepid "oxyphiles" on Dr. Tom's High Altitude Adventure. Outfitted with Sequal Eclipse POCs and Nonin recording oximeters, and accompanied by several respiratory therapists, nurses, and members of industry, we boarded our Magical Mystery Tour bus in Denver at 5,000 feet.

The ride took us to Echo Lake in the Colorado mountains at an elevation of 10,600 feet. Our oximeter readings were checked every 1,000 feet of ascent. This expedition was to evaluate the performance of the Eclipse. All of the oxyphiles fared well with pulse dose delivery, although one who was not accustomed to pulse dose O2 delivery did have to have continuous flow at the higher altitude. A festive lunch at El Rancho in Evergreen capped our successful adventure.

My next experience with the newly introduced POCs was a flight to Las Vegas using the AirSep FreeStyle in order to attend the 2006 American Association for Respiratory Care (AARC) Congress in December. I found the FreeStyle well suited to my oxygen needs during flight and continue to use it for air travel.

Registries and studies

In 2007 the COPD Foundation, with National Jewish Health, established the COPD Research Registry, a confidential database of individuals diagnosed with COPD or at risk of developing COPD. The registry was established to help researchers learn more about COPD and to help people interested in COPD research, find opportunities to participate.

The registry operates under the direction of the COPD Foundation's board of directors and is guided by an Oversight Committee comprised of leaders in the medical, ethical, scientific, and COPD communities. The COPD Foundation is working to ensure strictest confidentiality of participants. Information about the COPD Research Registry can be obtained by calling the C.O.P.D. Information Line at: 1-866-316-COPD (2673).

The vision for the COPDGene® Study was realized by Dr. James Crapo of National Jewish Health and Dr. Edwin Silverman of Harvard University's Brigham and Women's Hospital in Boston, MA. Subject recruitment began on January 1, 2008. It has 21 clinical sites throughout the country ranging from UCLA in California to Duke University in North Carolina. Complete information can be found on the Internet at the COPDGene® web site: http://www.copdgene.org/.

The COPD Foundation established a COPD Research Database in 2008. The web site is located at http://research.copdfoundation.org/ and includes a searchable dataset containing comprehensive information on a network of researchers, titles of research projects in COPD conducted since 2008, and locations of COPD focused research. You will also find links to related research resources such as patient registries, scientific and lay organizations, and publications and funding sources.

The mission continues

The National Heart, Lung and Blood Institute's Learn More Breathe Better Campaign was launched on January 18, 2008, in Washington, DC, with the purpose of spreading awareness of COPD. This campaign provides a full spectrum of print materials for both patients and professionals, along with extensive information on the web site: www.nhlbi.nih.gov/health/public/lung/copd/.

The American Lung Association of Colorado, the University of Colorado, and Colorado COPD Connection continued their tradition of leadership in lung health education with the first in a series of forums entitled "Breathing Matters; Living Well With Chronic Lung Disease" at the University of Colorado Hospital in August of 2009.

Led by the ATS and the Forum of International Respiratory Societies, the "2010: The Year of the Lung" public awareness campaign officially launched on December 5, 2009, at the 40th Union World Conference on Lung Health, in Cancun, Mexico. On January 15, 2010, the American Lung Association of Colorado, the University of Colorado, and Colorado COPD Connection presented the first "2010: The Year of the Lung" event with a second "Breathing Matters; Living Well With Chronic Lung Disease" forum at the Native American Health Center on the Anschutz campus of the University of Colorado.

Singularly blessed

All of these programs, studies, and events are doing wonders for COPD awareness.

For myself, getting involved in COPD awareness and advocacy has provided me with a way to make a positive impact not only on my own condition, but on the lung health of everyone who comes away from the doctor's office with a diagnosis of COPD. Throughout it all I continue to "titrate as I migrate," (free download at http://www.perf2ndwind.org/html/tompetty/2006/Nov-2006.html) and thanks to Dr. Tom's legacy of LTOT, maintain a FEV1 between 35-40%. I consider myself singularly blessed with the privilege of representing and serving all of the patients, caregivers, and health care providers who deal with the day-to-day problems of living with a chronic lung disease.

My Journey Through the Wonderful World of COPD Advocacy

I was introduced to the world of respiratory conferences when I attended the 2006 American Association for Respiratory Care (AARC) Congress as editor of *Everything Respiratory* magazine. The experience provided me with the incentive to become active in national COPD Awareness activities:

I attended the National, Heart, Lung and Blood Institute (NHLBI) Public Information Organization (PIO) meeting in Bethesda, MD, as the representative for COPD-Alert in June 2007, followed by the October CHEST Conference in Chicago and the December AARC Congress in Orlando as a member of the COPD Foundation.

In 2007 I was appointed as a consultant to the Food and Drug Administration's Patient Representative Program for COPD.

I was elected to the National Home Oxygen Patients Association (NHOPA) board of directors in 2008. In May 2008 I attended the Colorado Society for Respiratory Care Conference in Keystone, CO, and in June the NHLBI PIO in Bethesda, MD, as the Colorado COPD Coalition representative.

I was appointed to the EFFORTS executive board in 2009 and represent EFFORTS on the local and national level.

In March of 2009 I traveled to Washington, DC, as patient representative member of the Colorado delegation of AARC Political Advocacy Contact Team (PACT) with Allen Wentworth, RRT, and Leigh Otto, RRT. Allen and Leigh put me into a wheelchair with my AirSep FreeStyle and off we went via the Metro to the offices of all nine Colorado members of Congress.

In May I represented EFFORTS at the American Thoracic Society Public Advisory Roundtable (ATS PAR) during the ATS International Conference in San Diego, CA. Two California EFFORTS members, Dale Swank of Rancho Bernardo and Kathy Townsend from Anaheim, joined me at the U.S. COPD Coalition meeting during this conference.

In June I represented EFFORTS at the ATS PAR and the NHLBI PIO meeting in Bethesda, MD, and in July I was appointed as the EFFORTS representative to the ATS PAR Council of Public Representatives. April Obholz of the American Lung Association, Allen Wentworth of the University of Colorado Respiratory Medicine Department, and I planned the first "Breathing Matters; Living Well with Chronic Lung Disease," a program for patients, professionals, and caregivers that was presented on August 27 at University Hospital on the Anschutz campus in Aurora, CO.

The Fifth Annual Colorado COPD Conference, now officially designated "The Thomas L. Petty Moving Mountains COPD Conference" was held on Saturday, October 3, 2009, at the Police Protective Association Events Center in Denver. The conference continues to attract patients, providers, and professionals for a day-long program of educational presentations and vendor exhibits. The Colorado COPD Connection presented U.S. Congresswoman Diana DeGette with a certificate of appreciation for her contributions to health issues in the U.S. House of Representatives. Rep. DeGette has become a member of the Congressional COPD Caucus. Senator Michael Bennet joined the Congressional COPD Caucus in January 2010.

In 2009 Jean Rommes, the newest member of the EFFORTS executive board, accompanied me to the 11th Annual American College of Chest Physicians (ACCP) Community Asthma and COPD Coalitions Symposium in San Diego, CA. Jean represented EFFORTS and I represented the Colorado COPD Coalition at the Poster Presentation following the symposium.

Led by the ATS and the Forum of International Respiratory Societies, the "2010: The Year of the Lung" public awareness campaign was officially launched on December 5, 2009, at the 40th Union World Conference on Lung Health in Cancun, Mexico. The aims and objectives are to raise awareness about the importance of lung health, generate social and political support for preventing and treating lung disease, and increase public and private funding for lung research. The first event was "Breathing Matters; Living Well With Chronic Lung Disease," presented by the American Lung Association of Colorado, the University of Colorado, and Colorado

COPD Connection at the Nighthorse Campbell Indian Health Center on the Anschutz Campus of the CU Medical Center on January 15, 2010.

On March 8, 2010, Allen Wentworth, Leigh Otto, and I, with my trusty AirSep FreeStyle, once again took part in the AARC PACT trip to Washington, DC, visiting all nine Colorado members of Congress, bringing to their attention the concerns of the respiratory community in Colorado and the nation.

Scholars have long known that fishing eventually turns men into philosophers. Unfortunately, it is almost impossible to buy decent tackle on a philosopher's salary.

Patrick F. McManus

Chapter 14

Emphysema Foundation
for Our Right to Survive (EFFORTS)

Linda Watson, President

The Emphysema Foundation for Our Right to Survive (EFFORTS) was formed in May of 1998 by Sharon Adkins, Mickey Wagner, and Gary Bain, along with a small group of patients who wanted to have an online support list and working group to promote advocacy for emphysema/ COPD. There were no online support groups that engaged in emphysema/COPD advocacy at the time. EFFORTS (which can be found at www.emphysema.net) was the first. This small group of about 30 people grew to 900 by the end of 2000, to 2000 by 2005, and has since become an international, online, all volunteer, support/advocacy organization of over 2400 people.

The first chore for EFFORTS was to create a web site with pertinent information on treatment, support, links, and research for our members and the public. In 1999, tobacco companies were being sued, and the use of state tobacco settlement funds was a major issue for us. Our members pushed their states to direct these funds towards disease education and awareness, diagnosis and research, and treatment, in addition to stop smoking campaigns. We felt that there were many anti-smoking groups active against the tobacco companies, while the disease side of the equation was overlooked and grossly underfunded. We tried to increase funds for research, awareness, and even medical needs.

We were not trying to deny the effect smoking had on our health, or refuse responsibility for our own actions. We acknowledged all of that, but at the same time we wanted emphysema/COPD to be treated as a disease and not just a side effect of smoking. This would mean giving emphysema/COPD the early and timely diagnosis, treatment, research, and patient support that all other diseases routinely get.

Some of our activities

Questioning the amounts spent on research for emphysema/COPD, which was and still is the fourth leading cause of death, led us to begin writing to the National Institutes of Health (NIH) to find out how research funds were allocated. This resulted in our becoming one of their Public Interest Organizations (PIO). Being a PIO put us in a position to learn more about clinical trials and research and how we could become more effective campaigners for increased research for emphysema/COPD.

We continue to participate in their PIO activities and are grateful for what we have learned, as well as for the changes we have seen over the years in increased monies for research and COPD awareness — especially the wonderful "Learn More Breathe Better" campaign sponsored by the National Heart, Lung and Blood Institute (NHLBI).

EFFORTS asks members to be involved in their own communities in any way they can, promoting youth tobacco prevention and increasing the spread of information about COPD. We encourage our members to go out in public wearing their oxygen. We have made t-shirts, printed bumper stickers, mailed brochures and put them in our doctors' offices, and written letters to the editor and anyone else we could think of.

We have also established our own online stop smoking group. Originally called "Non-smokers Under Construction," it has now evolved into "Quitsters," an online smoking cessation program of EFFORTS. We have a program called "Walkers" to promote exercise and "Funday," a list for socializing and having fun. Many of us have written about our experience with this disease and smoking, and posted these stories on our web site as an educational resource for students, patients, and family members. We have been told time and again to quit smoking by family members and medical professionals but nothing has the impact of hearing it from another patient in the same position.

Rallying for the cause

In 2000, members began talking about having a rally in Washington, DC, to draw attention to COPD and create some public awareness regarding the lack of resources for the emphysema/COPD patient. That May approximately 30 members and their families and friends trekked to Washington to sit on the Capitol steps, listen to speakers, and try to get the attention of our Congressional representatives. The temperature was in the 90s and patients were on the steps struggling to breathe while their families raced back and forth with ice to help them keep their temperatures under control and their oxygen at acceptable levels.

Many of the professional organizations involved in respiratory care sent speakers to the rally. Among them were the American Lung Association (www.lungusa.org) , the American Association for Respiratory Care (www.aarc.org), the American Thoracic Society (www.thoracic.org) , the American Cancer Society (www.cancer.org) , other involved organizations, durable medical equipment providers, and transplant patients.

The following two years we went to Washington again in May, drawing more patient participation each time. Despite the hardship of travelling with oxygen equipment and medications, members and their families made the effort to get there.

In 2003, instead of going to Washington by ourselves, we participated in the first U.S. COPD Coalition Conference in Arlington, VA. That meeting set the stage for a merger of pulmonary professionals and patients that continues to have impact today. Thirty-two members attended, bringing with them their stories of what emphysema/COPD is like from the patient's point of view.

Two of our members' stories were selected for oral presentation. One was Pat Crowe's "You Think of Air Differently When You Have To Carry It." Pat was an executive board member and web site manager. The other was Vera Frank's "The Personal Side of Living with COPD," presented by Ron Cook. Sadly, many of

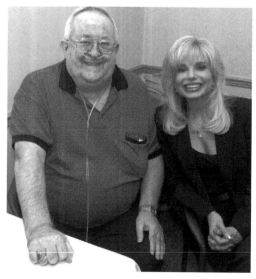

Gary Bain with actress Loni Anderson. Ms. Anderson lost both of her parents to COPD.

those who attended or sent abstracts, including Pat and Ron, are no longer with us to see the improvements that have been made.

My personal journey

I was first diagnosed in 1989. I came down with a very bad cold and went to our family doctor in my home town, even though his office was an hour away from where I was living at the time. He told me that I had COPD and I thought, "Thank God, I don't have emphysema." I was 38 at the time. I looked for information about this disease and could only find one book about emphysema at our local library. I thought, surely he means I will have this when I am 60 or 70, not now. Over the next ten years, I moved twice and had different insurance companies and saw several different doctors, this being the time when HMOs first came on the scene.

By 1997, I was having more severe, longer lasting bouts with bronchitis and was finally told that I had emphysema. I was prescribed an inhaled steroid, Atrovent, and albuterol, and tried to continue my life. At the time, I was still working part time, trying to keep up with the kids, their sports, and Boy Scouts, in addition to keeping everyone in clean clothes and fed. It was a struggle, with all this gasping for air going on.

In the back of my head, I still thought that I could exercise more, quit smoking, and get better. I didn't know that once your lung tissue is destroyed, there is no getting better. There is only the option of making better use out of what you have left.

Finally in December of 1998, I was able to quit smoking. That had been a ten-year struggle. I tried everything there was to try: hypnosis, the patch, SmokEnders, etc. It took continued attempts to finally succeed, along with a large dose of fear. It was getting harder and harder to walk and stairs were horrendous.

In the winter of 1998, my husband insisted on getting a computer. Finally, I had a source of information about my disease. I found a few web sites offering information and support. They were all good. I chose to remain with EFFORTS because they were the only group I had found that was willing to advocate for better treatment and research. I didn't want my children to suffer with this disease, as I had. I learned there were other people in the world who could not get across the room to answer the door;

some of them were even my age. I learned about all these new things: lung capacity, pulmonary rehab, and six minute walk tests. Things I had never heard of before.

Getting aggressive

It was finding EFFORTS that made me realize I could be more aggressive in getting treatment for my disease. In addition, a friend told me that my fingernails really should not be blue. We were back with a large insurance company now and I knew I had more options available to me. I knew I had to get to a pulmonologist. EFFORTS gave me the courage to pursue that track.

So back I went to my original family doctor. He immediately sent me to a pulmonologist at Mary Imogene Basset Hospital in Cooperstown, NY. After my pulmonary function test, the doctor and nurse came back into the office and told me my test results. He also gave me a prognosis of one to three years to live and prescribed oxygen. He discussed having an evaluation for a transplant, or possibly lung volume reduction surgery (LVRS), in order to extend my life.

I was in shock. The nurse was in tears. We had been talking about our boys, who were about the same age. At the time I was 49 and my youngest child was 10. But as awful as it sounds, it was exactly what I needed to hear. In all the years of going to doctors, I never had been given anything that I could use to judge the severity of my disease and understand what the implications were. Maybe I should have known, but I did not. I never saw anyone on oxygen and was only vaguely aware of emphysema as a disease. I thought it was extremely rare.

For some people, a diagnosis of emphysema means you don't want to leave the house because venturing out means a struggle to breathe. We keep trying to change that. I often get stopped by people who ask about this disease. Where did you get your oxygen and who diagnosed you and what can I do? I do think guilt keeps many people from seeking help. Some of my doctors had said you have adult onset asthma, some said chronic bronchitis. Since then, I have come to understand how unusual it is to be diagnosed in your thirties with emphysema. It is very hard to absorb all the information you need to learn about a disease in a 15 or 20 minute doctor's appointment, especially when that disease is a chronic disease. Slowing the progression of this disease requires education in nutrition, exercise, and smoking prevention.

Approved for LVRS

In 1999 I started the evaluation process that the pulmonologist had suggested at one hospital and my transplant was approved for either the Cleveland Clinic or Brigham and Women's Hospital in Boston. Then my husband's company decided to switch insurance carriers, and it was back to square one. The poor doctor had to start writing requests and filling out forms all over again.

We headed off to New York Presbyterian Hospital to finish the testing. I was approved and we decided to have the LVRS because it was possible that it would give me two to four more years before I would need a transplant. That was in June of 2000. It was a miracle that I was even able to have the surgery. I had just missed the National Emphysema Treatment Trial and the doctor had to convince the insurance company to pay for the surgery as it was not yet an approved procedure.

I first used oxygen in 1999 at the age of 47. My FEV_1 was .58 (L) and my percent predicted was 23%. I was prescribed two liters of oxygen for sleep. After the LVRS in 2000, I used oxygen for about six months, 24/7. This was my first daytime use of oxygen. After that, I was able to live oxygen-free for almost six years. I was able to see my son graduate from high school, which I wasn't sure I was going to be able to do back when he was 10.

Since there were no pulmonary rehabilitation facilities within 100 miles of my home, I bought an oximeter and started checking my oxygen saturation and exercised as best I could. My FEV_1 had gone up to .83 (L) and 33% two years after surgery. It was another four years before I went back on oxygen to exercise, in 2006.

At the age of 59, my FEV_1 percentage is now in the mid-teens. I use two liters to sleep and when sitting, and usually three liters for exercise. I do monitor my saturation with an oximeter and turn my oxygen up if I am attempting something more physically demanding than normal, such as carrying groceries uphill. My doctor is aware of this, and I always ask him if I have any problems. I now use liquid oxygen and prefer it. It allows for much greater mobility and the use of both hands, and is especially nice if you are a smaller person. I do use a backpack with my Marathon. Without it you are dragging a tank, or lugging a heavier compressed tank around. It's lighter than the portable tank I would need to stay mobile for the same amount of time. My shoulders appreciate it very much. I even use it around the house. A long hose connected to a concentrator can cause many spills and broken bones.

I have been on oxygen for the past three years now and have to decide whether or not to once again try for a transplant before I am too old to be considered.

EFFORTS continues to advocate and inform

EFFORTS' goals are still the same: to increase public awareness, to improve treatment and research, and to provide patients, their families, and caregivers access to information about their disease and support from fellow patients. The lack of information available to the public is still one of the largest hurdles we, as patients, have to overcome. I was amazed that I could have a disease that was the fourth leading cause of death in the United States, and yet there were no screening campaigns, no posters hanging in hospitals, and no educational or support programs available upon diagnosis, such as the type commonly provided for other chronic diseases. When I first joined EFFORTS I was astounded to learn about pulmonary rehab, and how important exercise is. I was thrilled to discover the Pulmonary Education and Research Foundation, the National Lung Health Education Program, and the COPD patient's hero, Dr. Thomas Petty. What did patients who did not have computers do for information, especially those in rural areas?

Since the formation of the U.S. COPD Coalition (see Chapter 13) and the COPD Congressional Caucus we have seen some basic improvements. We are now allowed to bring portable oxygen concentrators (POCs) on airlines. So we can fly without paying an extra $100 a leg for oxygen. We now have a law requiring Medicare to pay for pulmonary rehab for certain patients.

The NIH has increased funding for research as well, and we are extremely grateful to the NHLBI for establishing the "Learn More Breathe

Better" COPD awareness campaign. The World Health Organization, the Global Obstructive Lung Disease Coalition, and the International COPD Coalition continue to make advances, and we thank them along with all the other professional organizations that have stepped up to help. Many of these activities culminated in the first world conference of COPD patients held in Rome on June 14, 2009. I hope this trend continues and professional and medical organizations continue to join us as advocates.

However, there is still much left to do. We have yet to see the widespread use of spirometry screenings as a tool to monitor basic lung health. Although the COPD Foundation's Mobile Spirometry Unit is making great strides in promoting spirometry and early diagnosis, early and timely diagnosis that is routine for other diseases has yet to become the norm for COPD. Access to portable oxygen equipment is very uneven, and some patients have back-up equipment while others do not.

Following their example

As I said earlier, we are grateful for the strides that we and others have made in emphysema/COPD advocacy over the past decade. Much of our success can be attributed to some good friends we lost along the way, and in closing, I want to acknowledge two who had an especially large impact on our organization. Just this past year, we lost our long time president and founder, Gary Bain, as well as Frank Barrett, who had also been a member since 1999 and who served as vice president for most of those years. They gave endlessly of their time and energy.

We will do our best to follow their example and continue to provide information, hope, and advocacy to COPD patients, their friends, and families.

Chapter 15

Progress and Perspectives of Home Oxygen Therapy in Japan

Kozui Kida, MD, PhD*

Currently, the total number of patients receiving oxygen at home has reached approximately 150,000 in Japan. This was achieved in only a quarter of a century. Historically, oxygen therapy is clearly the leader and highly valued among several home-based care methods, such as the self-injection of insulin for diabetic patients or home-based dialysis for chronic renal failure. We are honored to support this therapy with the assistance of many medical doctors and health care professionals throughout the world.

An approach to oxygen therapy in Japan

The elderly population, aged 65 and older, is increasing in Japan, and is currently at its highest level ever: 28.10 million and 22.3% of the total population (2008). This increase in the elderly population will be further accelerated when the so-called 'baby boomers' reach retirement. By mid-century, the probability of having passed a specific aging threshold is 98% in Japan/Oceania, 82% in Western Europe, and even 69% in the China region. The increase in the size of the elderly population inevitably increases the number of patients with chronic illnesses, as well as the individual morbidity rate. A recent report (2009) from the USA indicated that Medicare beneficiaries with five or more chronic conditions accounted for 76% of Medicare expenditure. There are several unique characteristics of the system of medical insurance in Japan: all citizens have to join public medical insurance, all are entitled to free access to any medical institution using the insurance, and 70-90% of the direct medical costs are covered

* Dept. of Pulmonary Medicine, Infection, and Oncology; Respiratory Care Clinic, Nippon Medical School, Tokyo, Japan.

under it. In general, elderly patients have been mostly managed by local and larger hospitals in Japan, similar to younger patients using the same medical insurance. However, it was found that there was a problem on both sides regarding patients and their families or caregivers, and policy makers in terms of reimbursement. Therefore, a strategy was promoted to place home care as the core of the medical system for elderly patients. This was one reason for the progression of home care in Japan in the early 1980s; however, the reason was not only to reduce medical costs, but also to shift toward improving the quality of life of patients. This has been achieved through the application of modern technology. Reform or constant efforts to ensure more efficient and inexpensive home care for elderly patients continue. The Medical Service Law was revised in 1992, and the health care insurance system was implemented in 1994; nevertheless, increased costs in the future are unavoidable, and so a new insurance system for the old-old elderly (>75 years old) was started in 2008.

Historical view of home oxygen therapy in Japan — At the dawn of oxygen therapy

Respiratory care in Japan is currently progressing along with long-term oxygen therapy (LTOT). LTOT is more commonly called HOT (home oxygen therapy) in Japan by doctors, health care professionals, and patients. The abbreviation HOT was used firstly in 1981 by myself. I look back on it with nostalgia. At an annual meeting of the Japan Geriatric Society, I presented a paper regarding a clinical study of oxygen therapy in elderly patients. A chairman of the session, Dr. Michiyoshi Harasawa, a professor of medicine at Tokyo University School of Medicine, who passed away in 2002, made fun of me and asked "Is HOT correct English?" I replied "No, not at all. This is Japanese-English coined by me." However, since then, LTOT has been referred to as HOT in Japan. When I first used the term HOT, I imagined that HOT is opposite to COLD, which is a synonym of COPD (chronic obstructive pulmonary disease) and much easier to pronounce for Japanese compared to LTOT.

There are several reasons why HOT has become established in a relatively short period in Japan. First, the marked progression of medical technology in this area was realized. By the mid-1960s, Clark and John Severinghaus electrodes (thin needles) facilitated the clinical blood gas analysis of oxygen and dioxide. Pulse oximetry was discovered by accident by Dr. Takuo Aoyagi in Japan while trying to measure dye indicator cardiac output with an ear probe. The device (pulse oximeter) has been widely adopted as a standard for clinical measurement in the operating room, intensive care unit, and on the hospital floor, at rest, during wakefulness, or sleep. The development of oxygen concentrators and ambulatory oxygen systems has freed patients and caregivers from having to rely on bulky cylinders. Teijin Co., which is known for polymer chemistry, is one of the leading companies in this area. People of the Institute of Teijin applied a new technology involving a very thin membrane which is able to specifically separate oxygen from air. The membrane of the concentrator generates approximately 40% oxygen, which then passes through molecular sieve concentrators (>95% oxygen) that are used worldwide.

Reimbursement for home oxygen therapy

In 1985, HOT became covered by the public medical insurance in Japan. The medical insurance criteria for HOT are similar to those of other countries. However, initially, all patients who received HOT had to be reported to the local government, so that only chest specialists at large local hospitals were able to prescribe it. Therefore, the total number of patients was small. Then, this regulation was changed and general physicians who were working at all small hospitals or clinics were allowed to prescribe HOT. The total number slowly increased, since most of these small clinics do not have a blood gas analyzer, but the prescription is simple through maintaining a record of oxygen saturation using a pulse oximeter.

After acceptance of reimbursement

At the dawn of HOT in Japan, collaboration was encouraged between academic societies and industrial companies. There were groups such as the Japan Respiratory Society and Japan Society for Respiratory Care and Rehabilitation, and technology companies such as the Teijin Company in Japan. This collaboration promoted further progression after the acceptance of reimbursement for HOT. At the initial stage, however, HOT was performed only at large city hospitals after in-depth medical examinations. For example, it is unbelievable at present to think that some patients underwent right cardiac catheterization to clarify the presence of pulmonary hypertension, which was simply to decide on the indication for HOT. The number of patients receiving HOT increased but still remained low. In 1988, Dr. Thomas L. Petty, a professor at the University of Colorado in Denver, Colorado, and his colleague, Louise M. Nett, RN, RRT visited Japan to promote HOT. They gave lectures in five major cities, Tokyo, Sendai, Fukuoka, Hiroshima, and Osaka, speaking on the concept of HOT. Detailed information was provided on respiratory care based on their rich experience in Denver. Sizeable audiences, consisting of mainly chest specialists, gathered in each place, and they took this new information back to their medical schools or large hospitals. This markedly promoted the concept and skills among many physicians who had hesitated to adopt new treatments. They often had the misconception that oxygen use, except for in hospitals, such as home or ambulatory use, was hazardous and illegal since fire regulations forbade people to use oxygen at home. They could not ignore this, although this regulation was changed before 1988. After its promotion, an educational conference for both doctors and health care professionals was held every year at a small institute, at the foot of Mt. Fuji by Louise Nett and her colleagues, and we called it the Nett Conference. Dr. Toshihiko Haga, who was a director of the National Chest Hospital in Tokyo, was a key figure on the Japanese side. I worked with him as his assistant. This three-day conference was held annually for five years (1989-1993), and I attended every time. The members of the conference consisted of doctors and local health care professionals. It was very interesting and fun, and we learned how a team approach is important for HOT. These activities contributed to the subsequent progression, including the development of pulmonary rehabilitation and respiratory care in Japan. In February 1994, Tokyo Home Care for Respiratory Diseases was begun, and I have been its secretary general from that time to the present. Similar research groups started rapidly throughout Japan, numbering approximately more than 50 at present. Most of them are supported by chest physicians and health care professionals in local communities.

Development of comprehensive pulmonary rehabilitation in Japan

In 1994, I obtained a research grant from the Ministry of the Environment and became a chief of a research group. We decided to start a new project to study the benefit of HOT for pulmonary rehabilitation, as advocated by Dr. Petty and Louise Nett previously, involving an on-the-spot inspection for pulmonary rehabilitation as an initial stage. In January 1995, a total of 11 researchers visited three institutes in the USA. We first visited the Little Company of Mary Hospital in Los Angeles. Mary Burns, BS, RN, a director of nursing, kindly provided us with all information on comprehensive pulmonary rehabilitation, which was very impressive. It characterized a team approach and was well-organized, including nutrition and exercise for COPD patients. In those days, pulmonary rehabilitation in Japan was mainly achieved by physiotherapists alone, and they only guided patients in postural drainage or breathing techniques through diaphragm training with patients lying on their back. Neither pursed lip breathing on walking nor ways to improve activities of daily living were taught to patients with breathing difficulty. We met Dr. Richard Casaburi, a very well-known scientist in the field of pulmonary physiology, at Harbor-UCLA Medical Center in Los Angeles. I was deeply impressed to see research collaboration between the groups of Dr. Casaburi and Ms. Burns. Clearly, pulmonary rehabilitation is a practical application and the basic concept should be rooted in accurate science and up-to-date information. The former is like the leaves or beautiful blossoms of a large tree, and the latter is like a trunk or root of the tree. This idea has guided me in my research since then. We then visited St. Helena Hospital in San Francisco, where Dr. John E. Hodgkin provided us with a great deal of information connected with HOT and pulmonary rehabilitation from an academic perspective. I later contributed one chapter to a well-known text book edited by Drs. John E.Hodgkin, Bartolome R. Celli and Gerilynn Conners, BS RCP RRT, "Pulmonary Rehabilitation: Guidelines to Success, 3rd edition (2000)", on his invitation. Subsequently, we visited Kuakini Medical Center in Hawaii, which was originally established by Japanese immigrants. Medical staff including Mrs. Helen Ono, who passed away in 2000, and Ms. Kris Hara gave us useful information and details on the technology for HOT. Based on all this information, provided by many kind friends in the USA, I proposed a working hypothesis to combine HOT and comprehensive pulmonary rehabilitation. This concept is adopted in clinical guidelines by both the Japan Society for Respiratory Care (2003) and the Japan Respiratory Society (2005 and 2009). The hypothesis is mainly an instruction for patients with HOT and comprises seven different components, as follows:

1) all information needed in daily life such as on smoking cessation and ways to avoid acute exacerbations;
2) proper daily exercise at home;
3) proper nutrition to avoid obesity or losing too much weight;
4) taking medication on a regular basis, particularly for inhalations;
5) techniques to use oxygenation equipment for improved adherence and safety;
6) various pulmonary rehabilitation techniques such as pursed lips for breathing difficulty; and, finally,
7) self-management to maintain and increase social activity.

In order to facilitate all of these initial assessments by doctors and health care professionals regarding social activities and environments, as well as medical examinations are essential, since comprehensive pulmonary rehabilitation is based on science. If the hypothesis is correct, HOT could result in all patients achieving a better quality of life, decreasing the frequency of hospitalization and length of stay, or improving a depressive state. Based on this, we are pursuing various areas of clinical research, and publishing the results in academic journals, as well as providing detailed explanations in many text books for health care professionals, physicians, as well as for general citizens. I have always tried my best to disseminate useful information through the mass media, such as TV or radio programs, newspapers, or lectures, at various places. The research still continues at present, although the researchers have changed except for me. Two textbooks on pulmonary rehabilitation for health care professionals were published in 2003 and 2007, respectively, with collaboration by the Japan Respiratory Care and Pulmonary Rehabilitation and the Japan Respiratory Society. The first book is a manual for exercise and the second is for patient education on various respiratory diseases, particularly for patients with COPD. In 2008, I became a president of Japan Respiratory Care and Pulmonary Rehabilitation and held the annual conference in October 2009. The general thesis of the conference was "how we can achieve better patient education," and approximately 1,200 people gathered, presented papers, and discussed respiratory care.

The total number of respiratory physiotherapists reached approximately 18,000 in 2009. A new system for authorized nurses for respiratory care is expected to start in 2010 with the support of the Japan Nursing Association, and it will become central in respiratory care in the future as it will be advanced and very specialized for respiratory patients.

All this constitutes the history and progression of respiratory care in Japan. We are all aware that our starting point was HOT, and the achievements were facilitated by numerous people across many countries.

Current problems regarding oxygen therapy in Japan

With an attempt to increase awareness of the huge burden of respiratory diseases among the public and policy makers, the Japan Respiratory Society published a White Paper on a survey of home respiratory care in 2005. A total of 2,237 patients who belonged to the Japan Federation of Patient Organizations for Respiratory Diseases responded by post. Of those who returned the questionnaire, 55% were receiving HOT and/or home mechanical ventilation (HMV). COPD was the leading cause of disease (39%), followed by sequelae of pulmonary tuberculosis (35%), most of them were elderly, and they had complained of breathlessness or sputum production for a long time. Reasons for joining the patient advocacy group were that "they could get information about their disease and treatment" (75%), and that they "could learn about their disease" (81%). It was found that the activities of daily living of these subjects were restricted: 21% of those in the HOT/HMV group were home-bound, although 87% overall were not home-bound but their activities were severely restricted. The main reasons for restriction were inconvenience of ambulatory oxygen use (68%), fear of increasing dyspnea on leaving the home (63%), and solitude (50%). Regarding the economic burden, personal expenditure of these subjects reached more than 12,000 yen per month (120 US$) in 26% of the cases, which was similar in 46 and 31% of the HOT/HMV and HOT only groups, respectively.

Then, a survey of institutions accredited by the Japanese Respiratory Society, the Japan Physicians Association (mainly general physicians), and randomly selected general hospitals conducted in 2004 also appeared in the White Paper. Among various diseases, COPD is the leading disease (48%), followed by sequelae of pulmonary tuberculosis (18%), interstitial lung disease (15%), and lung cancer (5%). It is a characteristic that diseases treated by HOT differ from the USA, where most of the patients have COPD. From the survey on both patients and physicians who engaged in medical management, the following four areas were highlighted regarding the needs of patients: 1) improvement of the education and support for self-management; 2) approach to welfare; 3) creating a system of safe and anxiety-free home respiratory care; and 4) increase public awareness of respiratory diseases and patients with respiratory disabilities.

Problems in patients with COPD

COPD is characterized by symptoms of cough, sputum production, dyspnea, and exercise limitation. It is a common disease with an increasing prevalence, and currently is a major public health problem among elderly populations of developed countries including Japan. The global prevalence in adults aged >40 years is estimated to be 9-10%. Several problems among current issues are pointed out in patients with COPD. There are many under- diagnosed COPD patients. According to a report of the Ministry of Health, Labour and Welfare in 2005, the number was estimated at only approximately 220,000. However, an epidemiologic study on COPD performed in 2001 suggested that approximately 5.3 million Japanese aged 40 and older have COPD, and 15.7% of those aged 60 to 69 and 24.4% of those aged 70 and older. Further, it also showed that 1% of all COPD patients are in Stage IV (most severe), and HOT is generally administered for this stage based on recent clinical guidelines. The total number of patients receiving HOT is currently approximately 150,000, and about half of these are likely to suffer from COPD. These data suggest that only patients with the most severe COPD are likely to be picked up for proper treatment using HOT. Ironically, this may suggest that many physicians are more interested in expensive treatments or only severe cases. Therefore, only the tip of the iceberg is carefully being watched; there are many patients with severe COPD going undetected.

Previously, my colleagues and I reported the statistical analysis of a large series of autopsy cases at a large geriatric hospital where I was working for a long time. We studied comorbidity (complications) of emphysema (the extensive destruction of lung tissue) in elderly patients numbering of 4,553 cases, consisting of men (n=2,337) and women (n=2,216), with a mean age of 79.3. Since, traditionally, COPD comprises emphysema and chronic bronchitis, and is defined by airflow obstruction (functional abnormality), the level of emphysema indicates the severity of COPD after death. In this study, it was found that cerebrovascular disorder (brain infarction) is the leading comorbidity (complication) of elderly populations, being significantly more common than cases without emphysema. Although the incidence of coronary heart disease has been increasing recently, several reports suggest that the incidence of cerebrovascular disease is still higher in Japan or Asia compared with North America, in which heart disease is more common. Unfortunately, however, recent data indicate that the prevalence of heart disease is rapidly increasing among the younger generation. This is due to their preference for Western food rather than traditional Japanese food. Additionally, they exercise less while consuming high-energy foods. We learn from the observations that: 1) the prevalence of pathological emphysema with moderate or marked severity is very high, approximately 20%, in elderly patients; 2) a greater prevalence of lung cancer is noted in cases of severe emphysema, so that lung cancer is likely to be a complication of COPD; and 3) the total level of smoking (pack x years) is strongly correlated with the severity of emphysema. This provides a key message that COPD is not a simple lung disease, but may complicate various diseases as well. These include cardiovascular diseases, lung cancer, osteoporosis, muscle weakness and wasting, and depression. It is clear that all these are lifestyle-related diseases, and one common cause is a smoking habit.

It is only natural that people want to spend their last days comfortably. However, we found that this desire is lost on developing an unexpected illness such as COPD at an advanced age. We assessed the primary outcome by types of home care in elderly patients with COPD. The type of home care may be affected by various cultural or religious factors, since, in some

Asian countries, such as Korea or Japan, which are historically under Confucianism, families and relatives respect their elders and live together in a large house. The elderly were always treated respectfully by all family members, and they supervised the family with gentle eyes. However, currently the Asian style of caregiving is rapidly changing and being modified to the Western style due to difficulties in maintaining enough space to live together as a whole family. Many patients with HOT are in a difficult situation, because they cannot live together with their family. It is difficult for them to understand this at an advanced age.

Lessons from Japanese experience

Primary care is becoming increasingly focused on in the management of chronic disease in the health care system, and is more suited to episodic care of acute illness. Patients with chronic disease take more medications, see more specialists, and receive more formal and informal care. This is the nature of elderly patients with many chronic illnesses. For medical care of the elderly, information about the disease collected from younger adult patients is not always applicable. A wide range of information, extending from the changes associated with aging to the status of diseases of old age and health/well-being, must be sought. Medical care of the elderly should be holistic and comprehensive. Comprehensive respiratory rehabilitation adopts this concept, for which the United Nations designated the year of 1999 as the International Year of Older Persons, and promoted the Active Aging Initiative to facilitate active aging, devoid of diseases, and with only slight impairment, if any. In this process, five goals: independence, participation, care, self-actualization, and dignity, are specified. Medical care is closely involved in achieving each of these five goals. We have learned so many things from patients with HOT; however, unfortunately, the majority of them still wait for help.

Conclusions

At the initial stage, HOT was transported from the USA to Japan based on the efforts of many kind people. A quarter of a century has passed since HOT became covered by medical insurance, and the total number of HOT patients has reached approximately 150,000. About half of them are patients with COPD. This number is gradually increasing, although various efforts to tackle this have been made. We know that prevention is the best therapy, and so smoking cessation should be emphasized. Our experience through the development of HOT in Japan should be advanced by the next generation. In addition, information obtained should be disseminated to people in other countries. Medicine has been carried as a torchlight by many runners, and I feel privileged to have carried it a small part of the way.

"The charm of fishing is that it is the pursuit of what is elusive but attainable, a perpetual series of occasions for hope."

John Buchan

Chapter 16

Oxygen Use in Poland

Jan Zieliński, MD

History

The first written report on in-home oxygen use in Poland comes from the year 1926. Famous Polish poet and writer, Jan Kasprowicz, suffered from severe left heart failure and bouts of nocturnal pulmonary edema. The writer's wife, Maria, wrote in her diaries, "During the fourth attack, oxygen was used for the first time. This gave Johnny some relief. I told him not to be afraid of oxygen since similar was always used by Andzia`s (sister of Maria Kasprowicz) husband during his attacks of asthma."

My adventure with oxygen started in the 1960s when I was continuing my residency in internal medicine at the Institute of Tuberculosis in Warsaw. The name of the hospital was related to early post Second World War time when an epidemic of tuberculosis was ravaging Poland with 600 new cases per 100,000 population each year. To control tuberculosis, the Ministry of Health decided to create a special institution named Institute of Tuberculosis. This Institute was to organize a net of antituberculous out-patient clinics, where it would be possible to diagnose and isolate patients with tuberculosis in tuberculosis wards and antituberculosis sanatoriums. The patients would be treated and monitored given a nourishing diet and good mountain air.

In the1960s there was much less tuberculosis in the country. As a result, the Institute took care of other lung diseases arising from any patients admitted to the internal medicine part of the hospital. This was especially true in the winter time, when patients with chronic cough, purulent sputum, dyspnea, edema and other signs of the right heart failure were admitted. They all had severe hypoxemia confirmed by a time consuming tonometric method. Examination of one arterial blood sample required 30 minutes. Patients were given oxygen to breathe via a nasal catheter. We quickly learned that oxygen has to be given at a very low (2-3 liter) flow. After a few hours of high flow (6-8 liters) of oxygen, the patient would go into a respiratory coma.

The most spectacular effect of oxygen was a profound diuresis and quick recovery. Then the patient was able to perform spirometry which, at that time, was called spirography. Lung volumes and flows were measured from breathing maneuvers traced on calibrated millimeter paper. Spirography confirmed severe airway obstruction. Diagnosis of chronic bronchitis, respiratory failure, and cor pulmonale was established. When the patient was ready for discharge there was still one disturbing sign. The patient remained hypoxemic. In two or three months, the patient was back in the hospital with the same clinical picture as at the first admission.

It seemed that assuring a hypoxemic patient's possibility to breathe oxygen continuously at home would prevent recurrent deteriorations. Some patients took initiative to install heavy steel oxygen cylinders in their homes. Doctors could not prescribe oxygen for home use because the fire department did not allow residents to keep pressurized oxygen at home for risk of explosion. Soon, reports from Denver by Dr. Tom Petty and colleagues published in scientific journals objectively confirmed our bedside observations.

However, it was only after the milestone of controlled trials on effects of long-term oxygen treatment in patients with COPD (known all over the world as the Nocturnal Oxygen Therapy Trial (NOTT) and Medical Research Council (MRC) trials) a rationale was provided for routine use of long-term home oxygen treatment (LTOT) to treat respiratory failure.

The 1980s was a very frustrating period for us. At that time Poland belonged to a block of communist countries, which had been the case since 1945. In that system every citizen came under state health and social security, but the health care budget had no funds for new methods of treatment. The Ministry of Health remained unresponsive to appeals by the medical community to introduce LTOT.

In May 1985, I paid a short visit to Great Britain to determine suitability for Poland of two sources of oxygen used in the British Medical Research Council (MRC) trial. In the Birmingham area (Professor John Bishop) patients had been using a stationary source – oxygen concentrator. In Edinburgh (Professor David Flenley) patients were supplied with liquid oxygen. Although local technicians in Birmingham were worried by the high failure rate of early models of oxygen concentrators, Professor Flenley was very enthusiastic about the liquid oxygen system. There was no doubt that in Poland we should start with a more economic stationary source. That was my report to our health authorities. Shortly thereafter in Poland the decision was made to start LTOT.

To be well prepared, I applied for and was granted a two-week scholarship from the US Fulbright Foundation to visit Dr. Thomas L. Petty, Professor of Medicine at the University of Colorado in Denver, Colorado. Dr. Petty was the foremost pioneer of and expert in LTOT in the world. My visit to Denver in May 1986 was very fruitful. Apart from long discussions on LTOT with Dr. Petty, I participated in an anti-smoking course directed by Louise Nett, RN, RRT. I still keep an anti-smoking tie offered to me by Louise when the course was completed. I wear that tie when speaking on smoking cessation. The second week of my Scholarship I spent in Torrance, California, visiting the Research Laboratory for Exercise Testing directed by Professor Karlman Wasserman, where I met Dr. Richard Casaburi. An added and very appreciated bonus was to visit with Mary Burns, BS, RN, at the Little Company of Mary Hospital in Torrance. She taught me the basic knowledge of modern pulmonary rehabilitation.

In the fall of 1986, the Ministry of Health in Poland approved LTOT as a method of treatment of severe chronic respiratory failure. The Institute of Tuberculosis was charged with implementation of the system.

Organization

Between 1987 and 1991, the system was implemented nationwide. It was decided to incorporate an LTOT organization into a net of TB and pulmonary diseases clinics.

National guidelines were issued for indications for LTOT and the unified follow-up and care of patients undergoing LTOT. All physicians responsible for LTOT at a provincial level were trained at the Institute, and use uniform inclusion and follow-up forms. Physicians working at provincial LTOT centers have been certified pulmonary specialists.

Eligibility Criteria

The patients who qualified for LTOT were suffering from chronic respiratory disease leading to chronic respiratory failure. The main qualifying criterion is oxygen partial pressure in arterial blood lower or equal to 55 mmHg. The stability of the patient's status should be confirmed by two measurements performed 4 weeks apart. Also, patients with less severe hypoxemia, PaO2 between 56 and 60 mmHg, may be qualified for LTOT if their hypoxemia is accompanied by any two of the following signs:

1. Signs of pulmonary hypertension on a chest radiograph
2. Signs of a right ventricle hypertrophy on ECG
3. Elevated hematocrit, > 55%
4. Respiratory patients in whom severe hypoxemia was first diagnosed during hospital admission and remained hypoxemic at discharge are prescribed oxygen for three months. After that time a LTOT center makes the final decision about continuation or withdrawal of oxygen depending on results of blood gas examinations.

Patients with hypoxemia caused by heart disease or malignancy are not qualified for LTOT. For them oxygen may be prescribed as a palliative treatment by another branch of home care – palliative care and support. Patients who continue to smoke are also not qualified. The non-smoking status is verified by carbon monoxide measurements in the exhaled air. We do not prescribe LTOT for smokers for two reasons. First, because the elevated carboxyhemoglobin level in smokers reduces oxygen transport to the tissues. In the situation of insufficient resources, we would like to offer treatment to those who benefit the most. Secondly, smokers are at risk of burns when smoking cigarettes while breathing oxygen. Although a non-smoking condition is respected at entry, about 10% of the patients undergoing LTOT later resume smoking.

Equipment

The LTOT system in Poland is based on oxygen concentrators (OC). Several models manufactured in the US have been used during the last 20 years. In the years 1986-1998 OCs have been purchased by local LTOT centers and given to patients free of charge. Installation and maintenance of equipment was also a responsibility of LTOT center. That was very cumbersome for us. Since 1999 the national health system is financed by the National Health Fund (NHF), a stated-owned insurance company. Authorized dealers of equipment having contracts with NHF are notified about a new patient qualified for LTOT by the LTOT center. The dealer is responsible for installation and maintenance of equipment.

Follow-up

Patients undergoing LTOT are closely followed. They are seen at the LTOT center every three months. Every 12 months blood gases, spirometry, chest radiography, ECG, and blood count and hematocrit are repeated.

Patients unable to visit the LTOT center are visited at home by a nurse from the LTOT center. She assesses the general status of the patient, checks on daily oxygen use, and encourages the patient to use more oxygen if the oxygen-breathing hours are less than 15 per day. The oxygenation of the patient is assessed by a pulse oximetry method with the patient breathing oxygen at the prescribed flow. The reports are sent to a physician working at the center. We found that the nurse plays a crucial role in the system. As part of the professional medical workup, the nurse also helps patients with social problems and sometimes is the only caring person contacting lonely patients.

Patients Treated

Originally around 70% of patients receiving LTOT were patients with chronic obstructive pulmonary disease (COPD). Next in number were patients with post TB widespread pulmonary changes. Usually those patients presented also with signs of COPD. During the last few years the number of patients with TB sequelae diminished, and a number of patients with COPD increased to 85% of the total treated with LTOT in Poland.

Benefits of the System

The main benefit of the system is an accurate qualification procedure. This was and still is especially important considering insufficient funds allocated for LTOT equipment. Accuracy of qualification was verified in some 400 patients in 12 provincial centers. It confirmed a very high rate of accurate qualification. We believe that this very good result is due to the fact that qualification is assured by a specifically trained and instructed pulmonary specialist.

Another important benefit seems to be an opportunity to study large non-selected and closely followed-up groups of patients. We were able to perform original studies adding new data of importance to a daily practice of LTOT. One of the important questions we tried to answer was: should LTOT be withdrawn from a patient in whom, on consecutive follow-up measurements, PaO2 is above qualification level? We followed a group of 400 patients for at least three years looking for evolution of PaO2 under treatment. We found that in patients qualified for LTOT, improvement of PaO2 above qualification level was very rare and transitory. The further course of the disease in those patients was similar to patients in whom PaO2 steadily deteriorated.

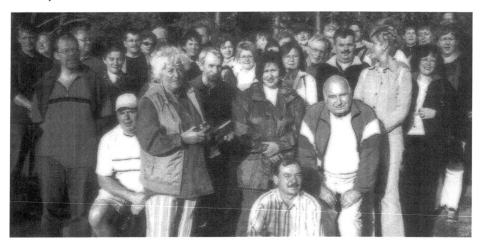

LTOT conference; Miedzyzdroje

Other original investigations were prospective longitudinal observations of effects of LTOT on pulmonary hemodynamics. This was the longest and largest study published so far on that topic. It was found that LTOT, after initial reduction of pulmonary hypertension, stabilized pulmonary arterial pressure over six years despite deterioration in arterial oxygen pressure and increase in arterial carbon dioxide pressure.

The number of patients undergoing LTOT in Poland is slowly increasing. However, the total number is insufficient when related to needs. In 2008, in 60 LTOT centers there were around 6000 patients profiting from LTOT. This number gives an index of 15 patients on LTOT per 100,000 population. Such index is probably one of the lowest among European countries and members of the European Community.

Another weak point of the system is almost total absence of ambulatory oxygen. Only in one province of the country (Kujawy-Pomerania province) a contract was signed for providing patients stationary oxygen (oxygen concentrator) or liquid oxygen with ambulatory oxygen canister.

Ambulatory oxygen devices – liquid oxygen and variety of portable oxygen concentrators are available for purchase from companies selling equipment for oxygen treatment. However, very few patients can afford such devices.

Team Spirit and Friendship

Since the very beginning of the home oxygen system in Poland, physicians working at provincial LTOT centers meet together each year for a one and one-half day conference. During the conference new developments in equipment and accessories for LTOT are presented. New indications for LTOT proposed by international panels of experts and characteristics of LTOT in other countries are discussed. Ample time is reserved for free discussion on local problems and joint policy towards National Health Fund authorities. The conference is organized by one of LTOT centers in the coun-

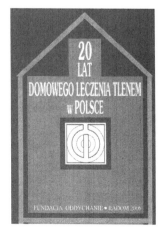

LTOT 20th Anniversary book

try, so each year it is held in different locality attractive to tourists. During more than 20 years, physicians working at LTOT centers have become friends with strong professional ties. Some pioneers of LTOT who retired, like the author of this review, continue to attend annual conferences to meet old and new friends. On 20th anniversary of LTOT in Poland a book describing the work of more than 60 LTOT centers in the country was edited and published.

We continue to look to the future for newer systems of LTOT. It is well known that patients prescribed stationary home oxygen become less physically active than before, mostly to comply with the prescription of breathing oxygen at least 15 hours per day. To prevent inactivity and deconditioning we investigate effects of simultaneous installation of home oxygen with a home-based simple rehabilitation program. We believe that improvement in exercise capacity by physical training while breathing oxygen may result in higher activity of patients, compared with not using oxygen. Mastering dyspnea during the rehabilitation period may encourage patients to attempt brief periods of outdoor activity with no oxygen supplementation.

"The greatest fishing secret ever?
Patience."
Donald Anderson

Chapter 17

Getting to Bibione

Giovanna Pizzi and Grazia Amoruso Banal

It all started when it was suggested that we travel from Milan, Italy, to Bibione, Italy, on behalf of the AMOR (Associazione Milanese di Ossigeno-ventiloterapia e Riabilitazione) to observe a typical day in the life of patients living with oxygen and to take part in a conference on the quality of life of people with respiratory problems who are on oxygen. As two people on oxygen ourselves, we were excited to make the trip. Little did we know it would be such an adventure!

The Blue Card

Although we are both on oxygen, we felt fairly comfortable making the trip by ourselves. A patient on oxygen therapy with a recognized 100% handicap can obtain a pre-booked ticket by calling Milan-Central station a few days before departure. On payment of a small fee, the ticket will be delivered directly to the home address, as long as the address is in the city of Milan.

The railways also offer companion service to those holding a Blue Card. These cards are obtainable upon presentation of a photocopy of the handicap certificate and a small payment. The Blue Card affords a discount on the ticket price of the patient and the patient's companion and his/her baggage to the train carriage. The service must be pre-booked by telephone on the day prior to travel.

We had heard that the National Railway offered a service to disabled people whereby they would be given help with baggage and, if necessary, help to their pre-booked seats on the train. However, we did not know it was only available to those who have a Blue Card. So on this occasion we had to manage by ourselves, with the help of a friend who had driven us to the station.

Of course, that meant that we had to leave the car parked where we risked getting a fine because there were no disabled parking spaces available in the vicinity. A railway official told us that such spaces had not been provided because the companion service was available — but, as already noted, it would take a Blue Card to get the service. So what now? As the saying goes, get yourself on the tram — or in our case, the train.

The usual curiosity

Despite these little glitches at the train station, we were looking forward to a lovely adventure: four hours of travel (depending on the proverbial Italian punctuality). All by ourselves, we were on the way to Bibione. Some might say "how reckless," but we had made our decision. We had undertaken this adventure, and only in the case of absolute necessity would we have changed our minds. We each had a suitcase and two full liquid oxygen portables, enough to meet our oxygen prescription requirements until we reached our destination.

Our departure time was 12:05. Now we were alone, except for our oxygen and cell phone for emergencies. We had only ourselves to rely upon, without panicking. The people in our carriage were full of curiosity, and there were some rather perplexed faces among them. Some whispered, "It's oxygen . . . oh no, it's something else" and "Imagine going around like that. It is a bit foolhardy." But after our fellow travelers' initial reservations, the journey turned into one of pleasant conversation with the people around us.

Three smiles

At 4 p.m. we arrived at Portogruaro. The ticket inspector had unloaded our baggage and very soon three members of ALIR (Associazione per la Lotta contro l'Insuficienza Respiratoria) from Vicenza arrived with two full liquid oxygen portables. We were very tired, but the sweet smile of Ines, the mischievous one of Luciana, and the placid one of Maurizio immediately put us at our ease. Within an hour we arrived at last at the hotel in Bibione, proud and happy with what we had been able to do.

The ALIR group consisted of about 30 patients with accompanying relatives, and they all gave us an enthusiastic welcome and immediately made us members of their work group. Ines, the nurse and group coordinator, explained to us that as well as the normal supply of oxygen, USSL (the national health service in Italy) could provide a "home hospital" service to patients who showed signs of recurring attacks of bronchitis or other illnesses that could be treated in familiar surroundings, thus avoiding unnecessary stays in the hospital. Medicines and other necessities are supplied directly from USSL. The whole project is coordinated by a team of doctors (Drs. Grison, Zanchetta, and Didone) together with a psychologist, a physiotherapist, and several nurses. The same team organizes one-week annual residential stays.

The start of the residential course

Everyday of the course we attended in Bibione was organized on the basis of standard criteria:

Physiotherapy: Individual exercises as recommended by the doctor.

Group therapy: Special exercises carried out in groups (muscles relaxation; exercises for the diaphragm and to help with expectoration, inhalation, and exhalation; and vascular fitness exercises.)

Psychological support: Relaxation exercises were carried out in small groups. This technique also helps those not suffering from respiratory problems and is offered by USSL of Vicenza to all who wish it.

Entertainment. Everyday there were periods of entertainment such as tombola (a family game similar to bingo), lottery, card games, and musical evenings with dancing (breath permitting).

The roundtable

Our time in Bibione was very significant. We didn't even notice the time passing, and every moment of the day we were conscious of feelings of internal well-being. We felt ourselves to be "two of them" and not guests. The time passed very serenely.

On Friday, Dr. Italo Brambilla arrived to take part in a roundtable with the moderator, Dr. Sala; the health director of USSL of Vicenza, Dr. Campedelli; chief of the department of rehabilitation, Dr. Caldana; and Drs. Mondini, Grison, and Zanchetta.

Dr. Brambilla is recognized for pioneering liquid oxygen in Italy and as such his lecture was much appreciated. According to the physician, successive meetings have confronted various matters connected with the organization of home-based oxygen therapy, with particular reference not only to local problems but also to legislative problems regarding respiration and the whole health system.

Among other things, one of the major problems was the lack of standardization of connectors for filling the portable oxygen containers. Thanks to these meetings, manufacturers must now provide compatible equipment.

We can do it!

Our trip to this conference of oxygen patients and health care professionals in Bibione was an experience neither of us will soon forget. Not only did we meet many other people who depend on oxygen just as we do, we proved to ourselves that we can travel with our oxygen, even when the circumstances are less than ideal!

A Cautionary Tale

Dr. Italo Brambilla

People on long-term oxygen therapy (LTOT) have always faced an uphill battle when trying to travel, and traveling by air has posed the worst problems. The following scenario is based on the real experiences of an Italian family in 2009. As you'll see, the road they traveled to get on the airplane was pretty rough. But they didn't let the obstacles keep them grounded.

The patient is Elena from Milan, Italy, who suffers from severe respiratory disease and requires supplemental oxygen. She wanted to travel by air because it was the only realistic way for her to complete a 1500 Km (1000 miles) roundtrip from Milan to Catania. The airline company was Alitalia.

Elena's daughter, a physiotherapist, booked the flight on May 1, three months prior to their departure. The departing flight was scheduled for 11:20 a.m. on August 6, and the return flight for 9:05 a.m. on August 24. A total of three tickets were purchased: a roundtrip ticket for Elena at 256.30 euros, a roundtrip ticket for the oxygen at 540 euros, and a roundtrip ticket for her daughter.

The airline company asked Elena's daughter to download a copy of the MEDIF form (required for travel with oxygen) and wanted to know who would be available to assist her mother and whether her mother's oxygen would be purchased by Elena or provided by the airline company. She was also informed that a certificate of identity signed by her mother's doctor would be necessary. Then she was advised to wait for a call from the Alitalia assistance office, which should come by May 4 or 5.

The phone call never arrived!

Due to the silence of the airline company, Elena's daughter called at the end of May and again in mid-June, receiving this response. "It is too early; you have to wait."

The family called the airline company three times on June 23 and received the same answer. "It is too early. We will call you."

On July 10 the airline finally called the family, denying the oxygen responsibility because they had too many passengers to carry.

The family sought help from the press, the Italian respiratory organization AMOR, and two physicians, Drs. Chiumello and Berardinelli. In addition, they wrote to the Alitalia public relations office and once again called the airline, asking if they would be allowed to travel if they chose different dates.

Finally the airline told them they could travel with different dates — and prices. The new price was 358 euros for the roundtrip passenger tickets. On July 20, the airline company called the family and confirmed the reservation. But it refused to supply the oxygen!

The family was advised to file a charge against the airline company for discrimination and failing to help a patient. Alitalia learned of the report and, fearing bad publicity, finally offered a solution: a portable oxygen concentrator (POC). The company said the family could choose between seven different types of this machine.

Elena's daughter made several calls trying to track down one of the machines for her mother to use on the flights. The Italian Medicare office ultimately agreed to provide an AirSep Free Style with a three-month rental at 450 euros.

On July 23 the family faxed all the documents to the airline company, and after many phone calls, Alitalia finally agreed to the flight with the POC.

Elena did fly, but at difficult and unreasonable hours for a patient, departing at 5 a.m. for both her Milan-Catania and Catania-Milan flights.

The morale of this story? People on oxygen will continue to fly, despite the roadblocks they face along the way!

"When there are no fish in one spot, cast your hook in another."
Chinese proverb

Chapter 18

The Role of the Respiratory Therapist in Home Oxygen Therapy

Mark W. Mangus, Sr., BSRC, RRT, RPFT, RCP, FAARC

Challenges and Opportunities

It would be difficult to complete this book without including a discussion of how Respiratory Therapists (RTs) fit into the long term oxygen therapy (LTOT) picture. While others have spoken about their experiences and *adventures* with oxygen, somewhere within that experience was an RT, whether cast in a prominent role or acting in one less visible. RTs can be spotted across the spectrum of health care delivery where the intervention of supplemental oxygen therapy is concerned. But, what they do and what they *should* do may be two quite different things.

Let's start by noting that RTs were born out of the advent of oxygen therapy in the hospital some 65 and more years ago! So, we began with and have developed around the vary core of oxygen therapy. Along the way we have been directed to other paths. Today oxygen therapy represents only one of our efforts. RTs are uniquely positioned to play a key role in identifying patients who need to use oxygen therapy. We are educated to be able to identify those who may need oxygen among those we encounter in the community. We are also well suited to be a primary source of information on oxygen use and to help users achieve optimal results with their use of oxygen. As staff members of pulmonary rehabilitation programs and physician practice settings, in addition to being employees of home medical equipment companies, we are on the medical care front line. Through affiliations with Better Breathers' Clubs and other organizations, we have the opportunity to play a broader role in educating oxygen users, health care professionals, and the public about LTOT. Exactly what role we can play and how we fit into the LTOT picture in the long run is limited more by our imagination and initiative than by opportunity.

Identifying those who need Long Term Oxygen Therapy

In a recent study of hospitalized patients with respiratory disease and who had hypoxemia, less than 40% go home with oxygen therapy despite demonstrating the continued need for it. Physicians and nurses can too easily overlook the needs of patients with chronic hypoxemia (low oxygen levels in the blood). Patients need the piece of the acute care puzzle that is our focus on the respiratory needs of the patient. Not only can we make the effort to assure that oxygen needs during the acute phase of patients' illnesses are appropriately met, but we can assess their ongoing oxygen needs after discharge. Only through our concerted effort to better identify those who have oxygen deficits can we drive intervention to correct them and more importantly, have a direct impact on improving the sad statistic mentioned a moment ago.

Effective RT intervention in the acute care setting must include methods to identify those who need oxygen therapy over a longer term. RTs need to be involved in discharge planning to help identify those who need to go home with oxygen. By working with discharge planners, we can help assure that those who need oxygen in the post-acute care setting receive it. We can assist with the selection of a system that most appropriately meets the home-care patient's needs. Our challenges here are to gain sufficient knowledge of oxygen systems and their advantages and limitations. We should help assure that what the home care patient receives from their supplier is both adequate and manageable, making adjustments as needs change.

Educating the LTOT User and Others

It is well documented that LTOT use has received a 'bad rap' through association with early use of oxygen therapy beyond the momentary supportive treatment for acute respiratory ailments. Not too many years ago, folks were prescribed oxygen therapy only when they had progressed to a severe disease state and were in need of it more for 'palliation' than for 'restoration'. Much effort has been spent over recent years trying to overcome the 'doom and gloom' perception, replacing it with a more realistic and positive one of oxygen as a therapy that 'enables' improvement in both health and quality of life. We have much work to do to further educate the greater public as well as the LTOT user to achieve this result while eliminating those outdated perceptions. But, we cannot stop there. Among the ranks of health care professionals, including physicians and nurses, there are many who continue to view LTOT with a jaded eye of doom and gloom. They hesitate to prescribe until hypoxemia is well advanced. They think those who exhibit moderate hypoxemia will somehow harden to dealing with their condition. They delay use of long term oxygen therapy. Many believe that by earlier institution of LTOT, users become dependent upon oxygen. As current evidence increasingly reveals, these notions are not only destructive, but are also based in false information, myth and conjecture. We have much to do to educate our healthcare colleagues to change any destructive notions about oxygen.

Evaluating those who may need LTOT

RTs are critical in evaluating patients for need of oxygen therapy and are able to do so through a number of methods and mechanisms. In the acute care setting, we have the tools of arterial blood gas measurement and pulse oximetry to directly assess and quantify oxygen deficits. While many measurements are necessarily made while the patient is at rest, we know that a person can exhibit adequate, even 'normal' saturation while at rest only to experience significant decrease and hypoxia when moving about. When able, they must be evaluated for ambulatory deficits and appropriate intervention. Again, in the process of discharge planning RTs need to intervene with assessment as the patient prepares to leave so that they are not discharged with hypoxemia that goes uncorrected. Evaluating prospective LTOT patients doesn't end with simply discovering who needs LTOT and prescribing the treatment. RTs need to help in the process of selecting the appropriate system and devices.

Walk tests to determine ongoing oxygen needs for ambulation must be a part of the process. Assessing activities of daily living to establish needs during their performance is another critical aspect. Learning what adjustments in oxygen delivery may be necessary and under what conditions they are needed is a key part of the process. Only through these actions can we successfully work to reduce the incidence of those cited in recent studies as going home without proper continuation of therapy. By instituting LTOT and reducing hypoxemia, we may avoid the complications associated with oxygen deficits.

Monitoring Those on LTOT and Making Adjustments

Once home oxygen therapy has been initiated, proper use of the system is necessary to assure optimal therapeutic benefit. RTs in home care settings are the best clinicians to help in selection and assessment of those devices to assure that they provide the best oxygenation possible under all conditions of use. Visits to measure oxygen saturation under conditions of use are in order at frequencies necessary to assure that each user makes best use of those devices selected for them or to make adjustments as necessary to accomplish that objective. Thereafter, periodic monitoring is necessary to assure that changes in oxygenation are met with adjustments in oxygen devices. RTs must continually hone their training and skills to meet the challenge of monitoring the patients. As technological advances produce new devices, RTs are challenged to become knowledgeable in the function and specifications of those oxygen delivery devices to be able to determine which ones will meet user's changing needs. Perhaps the greatest challenge to RTs today in regard to technological advancements is the sheer volume of knowledge required to sort out the differences between devices so as to know which ones are potentially suitable to address a given user's needs. This will be an unending process as the quest continues for production of devices that can do more with less and maintain practicality in terms of size and user friendliness.

Personal pulse oximeters are now smaller and less expensive than they have ever been, with some devices costing less than $100. These simple devices are easily understood by the average person. Dr. Petty often suggested to patients "To Titrate as You Migrate." In fact, he made this the subject of one of his Letters From Tom. You will find it at: http://www.perf2ndwind.org/html/tompetty/2006/Nov-2006.html .

Dr. Petty also wrote a booklet on personal oximeters, which is free for the downloading at: http://www.nonin.com/documents/go2/6965-000-01%20Dr%20Petty%20GO2%20Brochure_ENG.pdf

Challenges for the RT

While several challenges are evident in the previous paragraphs, it is appropriate to review those challenges as specific objectives toward ongoing and future actions on behalf of optimal LTOT therapy. To begin with, RTs in the acute care setting have undergone a shift in attention to and involvement with oxygen therapy. Owing to the perception that setting up, initiating, and managing oxygen therapy in the hospital is 'routine' and is lacking in complexity or difficulty, RTs are not always included. Ultimately little to no RT involvement may occur with its management. This lack of RT involvement can easily contribute to the statistic of patients who leave the hospital with continuing hypoxia that is not addressed with ongoing oxygen therapy. While the practicalities of administering and managing oxygen therapy may prohibit RTs from direct action to institute and manage oxygen therapy in the acute care setting, there are ways to keep RTs involved to better facilitate continuity of therapy beyond the hospital. This consideration could arguably be the most pressing short-coming in achieving more effective care of the broader population of those who can benefit from LTOT.

It is sadly apparent that RTs working in the acute care setting lack exposure to and knowledge of systems and devices utilized in LTOT. As a result, they lack understanding of how to determine home oxygen needs of patients who leave the hospital with ongoing supplemental oxygen requirements. While expectation to possess intricate and specific knowledge and understanding of the array of LTOT devices may be beyond the practical scope of the acute care RT, it is not unreasonable to expect them to acquire a basic understanding of types of home oxygen systems and their adjunctive equipment. This represents a most important challenge to RTs today and will remain so for the foreseeable future.

Gaps in knowledge and understanding of the technical capabilities of equipment used for LTOT have been identified among those working in the home care area; the very setting where such knowledge is most critically needed. While home care RTs may be restricted to using those devices that their employers purchase, they still are faced with the challenge to learn all they can about the capabilities and limitations of those devices. They should also learn about other devices that may better meet the needs of those they serve. By gaining the knowledge necessary to be effective in the selection of equipment they use, they will also become better teachers of those who use LTOT.

The Challenge for the LTOT User

While outlining and describing the various roles and challenges for RTs in supporting patients who use LTOT, there exist some notable challenges that include the patient as well. As mentioned earlier, many RTs do not possess the detailed knowledge necessary to best support LTOT users. While I admonish RTs who read this book and chapter to 'step up' and invest the time and effort to increase their knowledge and skill, let me also extend that message to patients using LTOT. Where those who would and should support you might fall short, you can and *must* take on the task *yourself* to learn all you reasonably can about the systems and devices you use as well as those that may hold possibility for increased benefit for your ongoing and changing needs. This is demonstrated by several of the patient chapters in this book. While you may not need to personally delve deeply into the technicalities of devices and advances, you *can* and *should* urge those RTs and others with whom you deal to make that effort. Don't be afraid to ask them questions that reveal their knowledge with regard to function and specifications of equipment. As you discover new devices or systems, ask your support team about them. You may find that *you* are the one who alerts *them* of devices and breakthroughs they had not stumbled across.

Another area where the street needs to be two-way is in self-monitoring of your oxygen needs. Many health care professionals who have a part in your LTOT experience are leery of the notion that patients can or should self-monitor and have their own pulse oximeters. As should be evident by this point in this book, we strongly advocate for patient ownership and use of oximetry. Just as a diabetic monitors his or her glucose to determine and adjust insulin doses, the LTOT user should do likewise in terms of oximetry to adjust oxygen dose. You as the patient can play a key role in educating *us* to come to understand the advantage in your self-monitoring activities. Only through collaboration can we gain comfort and confidence that this modus is indeed to the best advantage for all involved.

Keeping abreast of the latest and best in LTOT will continue to be a challenge for health care professionals like RTs *and* for you the user. By doing what you feel able and comfortable to do within the confines of your place on *your* LTOT 'team', you can enhance your experience while also sharing knowledge and experience with others. *You* can become the educator in many respects by challenging the RT to learn more about LTOT advancements.

A Few Closing Thoughts

RTs and others who are involved in administration and management of LTOT should realize and understand that they will be increasingly 'on notice' to step up to the challenges presented by the ongoing needs of all kinds in support of LTOT. The expanse of all that is involved in LTOT cannot be viewed and dealt with on a cursory basis any longer. It must continue to progress from an increasingly knowledgeable and organized point of view and modus operandi. LTOT is clearly a life-saving, life-sustaining and life-altering intervention. Meeting and conquering the many challenges facing the user and the RTs who serve them is imperative to its continued success. Effective LTOT requires a truly collaborative relationship between the user and RTs.

The Pulmonary Paper
PO Box 877
Ormond Beach, FL 32175
(800) 950 – 3698
Email: info@pulmonarypaper.org
Website: www.pulmonarypaper.org
ISSN 1047-9708

"The fishing was good; it was the catching that was bad."
K. Best

Chapter 19

Everything You Ever Wanted to Know about Your Home Oxygen

Robert McCoy, BS, RRT, FAARC

More than 225 years ago, English clergyman and chemist Joseph Priestley discovered oxygen by heating red mercuric oxide and capturing a colorless gas discharge. When he inhaled the gas, which he labeled "dephlogisticated air," he noticed a "light and easy feeling."

"Who can tell but that in time this pure air may become a fashionable article in luxury?" he remarked. That comment is not far from true. Today oxygen is not a luxury but a necessity for patients with some lung diseases.

Evolution of oxygen delivery

Oxygen delivery has evolved remarkably since Priestly made his discovery, with the most dramatic changes occurring in the past two decades. In the late 1970s, home oxygen concentrators began offering a more convenient method of providing stationary oxygen. Concentrators do not need regularly scheduled refills, which reduces the expense involved in visiting homes to refill oxygen systems.

Portable oxygen was first made available via the use of smaller cylinders. These systems usually weighed 20 lbs and required the use of a cart. In 1965, a liquid oxygen system (LOX) portable offered a lighter option with more operating range. LOX portables weighed approximately 8-10 lbs and could be carried by the patient. While these were great strides, weight and range-of-use remained big issues for most patients. Pulmonary diseases are debilitating, and any additional work related to carrying an oxygen system often countered the benefit of having portable oxygen to begin with. So lightweight carriers were designed for portability.

Conserving devices that efficiently use available oxygen are here to stay. While early systems were quite crude and bulky, the technology has evolved to be reliable, compact, and easy for a patient to use. Patients are no longer limited to staying in and around their homes; the development of oxygen conserving devices (OCDs) and the resulting technological advances have enabled them to have a longer range. This allows them to use their portable systems for a longer period of time.

Home oxygen benefits and limitations

Home oxygen equipment does not provide oxygen therapy. It is only the tool used by a knowledgeable person to accomplish appropriate oxygenation of a patient at all activity levels. There are many new options for home oxygen equipment that can address a changing market both for patients' needs and economic pressures.

The best new home oxygen system for a patient is the one that will keep that patient oxygenated at all activity levels. There are no home oxygen systems that can be considered appropriate for all patients. There is a significant amount of variability in performance capabilities between most products. Unfortunately, no standards have been developed for the amount of oxygen delivered by conserving devices or the maximum amount of oxygen provided by a portable oxygen concentrator, so each manufacturer has come up with its own capability requirements for its products.

Dose volume from a conserving device has been one of the challenging issues. Traditionally, the manufacturer determined the amount of oxygen delivered per setting (in ccs of oxygen) and labeled it equivalent to continuous flow at the same setting. This caused confusion, because when a patient did not oxygenate on one conserving device, the assumption was that the patient did not tolerate a conserving device and required continuous flow. If the patient would have been placed on a different conserving device, with a greater pulse volume, the patient might have been able to oxygenate and get the benefits of a longer lasting, lighter portable oxygen system. Oxygen conserving devices, when used appropriately with patient oxygenation as the outcome, can be a valuable tool for both the oxygen provider and the patient.

The unsophisticated approach of setting a dial on 2 and see what happens with patient oxygenation really isn't scientific, clinically effective, or appropriate. Most oxygen delivery systems are stagnate in the delivery of oxygen. This means that if the patient's demands increase, the product does not change its delivery of oxygen. Continuous flow blows a lot of oxygen past the patient's airways, and the amount of oxygen the patient receives as gas exchange units in the lung (alveoli) is dependent on inspiratory time, inspiratory flow rate, tidal volume, position in the inspiratory cycle for the delivery of the gas, dead space (delivery tubes in the lung that don't take part in gas exchange), and the fraction of inspired gas (FiO_2) from the delivery device. A knowledgeable clinician who can adjust the delivery of oxygen to a patient to give appropriate oxygen saturation during activity is the best way to conserve oxygen.

Selecting the right oxygen therapy equipment requires an understanding of a device's capability — i.e., how much oxygen it can deliver. A device that has the capability to supply a patient's needs at all activity levels is the right device. If the device is set on the highest setting and does not provide the minimum amounts of oxygen, it may not meet the needs of an active patient.

Patients want the lightest weight, longest lasting portable oxygen system out there. Home oxygen therapy has had a very poor compliance response from patients; they don't want to lug around a bulky, industrial looking oxygen system. These patients have a compromised pulmonary system, so a heavy portable is not feasible. Because conserving devices allow for a more efficient use of oxygen, lighter portable systems became a reality. Once again, conserving oxygen at the expense of oxygenation does not make sense. It will cost both the patient and the payer in the long run.

Home oxygen delivery is a more complex therapy than most clinicians realize. The rapid development of technology, clinical advancements, and economic pressures from payers have presented an educational challenge for all involved. Six Oxygen Consensus Conferences have been held over the past two decades to try to help all segments of the home oxygen industry understand and adapt to the ever changing issues.

What follows is an overview of the different components of home oxygen therapy.

Storage or generation of oxygen

Oxygen cylinders: Oxygen cylinders were one of the first methods of storing oxygen. Early cylinders were made of steel, and the regulators were typically made of brass. The combined weight of the cylinder, regulator, and cart was over 20 lbs, which made mobility with this type of system difficult. Today we have stainless steel or fiber wrapped cylinders, which can reduce the overall weight of portable oxygen cylinders. Cylinders come in all sizes, so they can be used for stationary or portable oxygen. Cylinders do not lose content when not in use, so are often used for emergency back up in any application where oxygen might be needed. Operating pressures are available in 2000 psi and 3000 psi. Each cylinder must be tested and labeled for the pressure used. The higher pressure cylinders can store more oxygen and can be almost as storage efficient as liquid oxygen. Cylinders used with home trans-filling systems have a safety mechanism in place to prevent an incompatible cylinder being filled from a trans-filling system.

Stationary oxygen concentrators: Since the early 1970s stationary oxygen concentrators have been the backbone of most home oxygen programs. The ability to generate oxygen in the home from an electric source has eliminated the need to continually refill package oxygen gas systems. These systems typically provide up to 5 liters per minute (lpm) of continuous flow oxygen, yet some systems have the capability to provide up to 10 lpm continuous flow oxygen. Oxygen concentrators generate approximately 93% oxygen +/- 3%; they are not able to filter out all trace gases that are found in the atmosphere. These units weigh between 30 and 50 lbs depending on the age and size of the unit. Therefore they are usually left in one location in the home. Oxygen tubing can be of a length necessary to provide oxygen throughout the home, yet caution is necessary to prevent tripping over the tubing, knocking items off of coffee tables, or tripping a family member. The length of the supply tubing will impact the flow of oxygen, so a liter meter is helpful to determine the actual flow of oxygen at the end of an extended length of tubing. Adjustments at the source flow meter can compensate for the length of tubing. Other issues related to stationary concentrators include:

Electrical consumption: This is based on the size and use of the stationary concentrator. Most home concentrators work at a constant workload, so the electrical usage is fairly consistent. The newer stationary concentrators have become more energy efficient, reducing the patient's cost of operation.

Noise: This is a variable issue depending on the patient's hearing level and the operation of the unit. Again, the newer units have become quieter, with some manufacturers offering units specially designed to be quieter.

Heat: All of the stationary concentrators will generate some heat due to their operation. Newer models have reduced the heat production as they reduce power consumption.

None of these issues have been significant, yet they need to be understood by the patient because they will be noticeable. Clinicians can easily explain them at the initiation of the stationary concentrator therapy.

Liquid oxygen systems

LOX has been popular for years and in use since 1965. It allows for a lightweight, long lasting portable system in which the patient can fill a single unit. The downside of LOX is that the provider needs to fill the base unit frequently, which is expensive because large trucks need to make frequent trips to the patient's home. Each step of the LOX delivery requires packaging, transfer, and monitoring, and each step has a cost associated with it. Additionally, LOX is always evaporating, which provides the operating pressure necessary to drive the oxygen flow yet creates the "use it or lose it" mentality with patients and providers. Large stationary oxygen systems are still used to refill a portable LOX system and are utilized for high flow oxygen demands. Stationary LOX units come in different sizes and are used to refill portables when the patient is traveling. Ten and 20 liter base units can be placed in the patient's care and provide a refill option for short trips where the patient wants to use his lightweight LOX portable.

Portable LOX became more popular with the introduction of a 3.5 lb system. This system changed the way home oxygen was provided. Patients asked for the product specifically and thus began to have a say regarding their home oxygen equipment. If a provider did not provide what the patient wanted, the patient would go to another provider. Patient service became an important part of provider services.

Liquid oxygen has the most efficient storage capability for packaged oxygen. Liquid oxygen has an expansion ratio of 860:1, meaning that one liter of liquid oxygen will expand to 860 liters of gaseous oxygen. This capability allowed for the longest lasting, lightest portable oxygen system. The introduction of conserving devices added to the operation time of a portable by efficiently delivering the oxygen during the patient's respiratory cycle. There are multiple sizes of LOX portables, with the smallest used mostly for shorter operation times and larger devices for longer operating times. High flow continuous oxygen is more efficient with LOX portables, again, as the package gas is more efficiently stored.

Stationary home oxygen systems that fill portables

Concentrators that fill compressed gas cylinders in the home are now available. Models differ between manufacturers, but the principles remain the same. A concentrator generates oxygen, then can transfer the oxygen as compressed gas into the portable cylinder. Oxygen monitoring equipment ensures the gas's purity. This allows patients to refill cylinders themselves, and it saves the home care provider from visiting the patient's home to exchange cylinders.

The cylinders are proprietary to each trans-filling system, so cylinders cannot be exchanged between different models or be confused with cylinders that are filled with 99% oxygen from industrial suppliers. At this time there are two levels of pressure available to fill the cylinders: 2000 psi and 3000 psi. The higher the pressure delivered to the cylinder, the more oxygen in the cylinder and the longer the operating time. Again, the cylinders cannot be exchanged for one another, so care must be taken to ensure the right cylinder is connected to the appropriate trans-fill system.

The patient only needs a few cylinders in the home and can fill the empty units as necessary, similar to a LOX system. These cylinders can be of any size. Patients do not need to worry about a small system not lasting for very long; they just refill the cylinder as needed. If more cylinders are needed for trips outside the house or vacations, the patient can request or purchase additional cylinders. Issues to be aware of with trans-filling systems include:

Purity of the gas is 93% +2/-3%: This less than 99% purity can be compensated with a slight bump in the liter flow or pulse setting if the patient is not at the top of the delivery range.

Pressure in the cylinder: Most cylinders are filled to 2000 psig, yet if the pressure is less than full, operating time will be impacted; 3000 psig cylinders allow for more gas storage with a slight increase in weight.

Oxygen conserving devices: OCDs have been an issue with all oxygen delivery systems, as each OCD provides a different pulse volume at a specific setting. Some of the devices drop the pulse volume as the patient's respiratory rate increases. If the OCD is integral to the cylinder (you can't change the OCD), and the patient cannot adequately oxygenate, especially with exercise, the entire trans-filling system will not be adequate for the patient and another system should be evaluated.

Increase in heat, noise, and electricity: The extra pumps on these systems will enhance the problems associated with concentrators in the home. The patient's individual situation should be evaluated to determine if this will be a significant burden. Some systems have separate pumps and may not have as significant an impact on the patient.

Fill times of the cylinders: Some systems are faster than others in filling portable cylinders, which is a marketing feature that can be attractive to the patient. The size of the cylinder is another factor that will impact fill time.

Oxygen concentrators that provide gas to a cryocooler that fills a liquid oxygen portable in the home have just become commercially available. Oxygen that is generated from a concentrator is sent to a cryocooler system and liquefied. This gas in not 99% pure gas, as some trace gases still get into the system and dilute the oxygen. These systems provide 94% oxygen in a liquid state.

The advantage of liquid oxygen is the weight to range benefit, as the

LOX has an 860:1 expansion ratio. Patients can get the benefit of a lightweight oxygen system, and the provider foregoes the expense of delivering bulk liquid oxygen. Liquid oxygen has the clinical benefit of a lightweight portable that encourages ambulation, plus high flow capabilities that may be necessary for oxygen patients with high demands. The issues to be aware of with home generating LOX systems are similar to those seen with home cylinder trans-filling systems.

Cylinder trans-filling systems

Small cylinders can be filled from larger cylinders. This technique has long been available for home care providers, yet was not available for patients to use in their homes until now. Large cylinders are readily available, and having patients trans-fill their own small cylinders at home means they can fill them as necessary rather than waiting for the provider to make a delivery. In addition to being more convenient for the patient, this is more cost effective too, because delivering oxygen is one of the most expensive services the provider incurs. The economics of home oxygen therapy spurred this trans-filling option. But be aware that not every patient is a candidate for trans-filling.

Portable oxygen concentrators

Portable oxygen concentrators (POC) were requested by attendees at the early Oxygen Consensus Conferences, who noted that ambulatory oxygen patients needed a better solution and a concentrator offered many benefits. These machines give patients the benefit of making oxygen where they are at rather than storing oxygen and carrying it with them. Even though the first POC was introduced in the mid 1990s it was not until a few years ago that several manufacturers introduced additional POC products.

The key to a POC is the efficient concentration and delivery of oxygen. All portables today use the same technology as the larger concentrators. The amount of oxygen concentrated in a minute is determined by the amount of sieve material (filtering material that removes nitrogen) available. A small amount of sieve will weigh less and produce less oxygen. A larger amount of sieve will produce more oxygen in a minute. The amount of oxygen produced in a minute determines the dose volume available at a range of settings. Less oxygen means a lower dose of oxygen per breath. The other factor is the POC makes a specific amount of oxygen in a minute. If the patient's breath rate increases, the POC cannot make more oxygen, so the purity of the gas may decrease. It is difficult to determine how a POC will work with individual patients unless the patient is tested on the device at all activity levels.

POCs have been a valuable addition to the options available for ambulatory patients. Making it easier to travel both by car and airline, they have allowed for extended times away from home with the option of plugging into any available electricity source. As such, they have provided a sense of freedom for patients who felt limited in their ability to travel.

On the flip side, the POCs have entered the market with very little research on their clinical capabilities, applications, and limitations. These devices work very differently than traditional oxygen delivery and most physicians are not aware of the issues. The systems produce less than pure oxygen, they use conserving devices, and they provide less oxygen as the patient increases his respiratory rate. With the lack of research and the lack of understanding of how the devices work, many patients are becoming the test pilots for providers and clinicians to learn how the equipment operates. This is not quite the best way to learn of medical product capabilities.

Issues to watch for with POCs include:

- Maximum oxygen production per minute.
- Oxygen dose per setting.
- How the device responds to increased respiratory rate.
- What affects the alarms and patient alerts.

There are currently two categories of POCs:

- Continuous flow capable with intermittent flow option, typically weighing approximately 20 lbs.
- Intermittent flow only, typically weighing 10 lbs or less.

Continuous flow POCs generate 3 lpm of oxygen. This amount of available gas allows the device to provide a large dose of oxygen when delivering pulse dose, as well as the option of continuous flow (CF). Patients with high oxygen demands have more options with the CF POC, as they can use the CF mode if the pulse is not meeting their needs, can use the CF mode with sleep if desired, and can bleed in the oxygen to another respiratory device (CPAP) if necessary. If a humidifier is desired, it can only be used with CF oxygen delivery, as the humidifier would interfere with the sensing device used with conserving devices.

Patients who need greater flexibility with their oxygen system find that the CF POCs can provide more options for higher oxygen delivery associated with increased activity and sleep. These units claim to have the potential to be both a stationary and portable system, and thus a single source for LTOT.

Intermittent flow POCs have a lower oxygen production and dose capability compared to CF POCs. These units are smaller and are easily moved, making them a natural first choice for patients. The smaller size also means less sieve material, so less capability to generate oxygen. Patients who have a lower demand for supplemental oxygen may benefit from these products. Lightweight POCs are ideal when engaging in minimal activity, such as flying in a plane, traveling in a car, or moving about in a wheelchair. The only effective means to determine if the POC is capable of a specific patient's application is to test with an oximeter. Clinicians should be involved in the initial assessment. A personal pulse oximeter is an effective tool for a knowledgeable patient.

Control of oxygen delivery

Continuous flow regulators and flow meters have been the standard for metering oxygen flow and are still the primary devices used in hospitals. The regulators control continuous flow and are very accurate and consistent. The devices do not react to the patient, so if the patient's breathing patterns or demand change, the devices continue to provide the set flow. This will be explained in more detail in the key issues section of this chapter.

Intermittent flow devices (conserving devices) have been developed to sense a patient's inspiratory effort and turn on a flow of oxygen for a defined time and then shut it off. Giving oxygen only when the patient is breathing is a more logical approach to oxygen therapy and provides a more accurate control of the delivered oxygen.

Many manufacturers are developing new methods of using oxygen conservation concepts and techniques to improve the response of their system in meeting the patient's constantly changing oxygen requirements due to their continually varying levels of activity. Methods utilized by an OCD to respond to a patient's changing oxygen needs include:

Pulse flow: Pulse flow is defined as the device responding to the patient's inspiratory effort and terminating flow at a predetermined time controlled by an electronic circuit board. Pulse systems typically need a power source, so batteries are a factor to consider.

Demand flow: Demand flow senses the patient's inspiratory effort, yet flow is terminated on exhalation. The amount of oxygen delivered will vary with inspiratory time. These units are not as efficient as pulse flow in utilization of oxygen, yet have the advantage of not requiring batteries. Most demand systems use a duel lumen cannula with one channel of the cannula sensing inspiration and the other channel delivering oxygen.

Respiratory rate regulated flow: This device monitors the patient's respiratory rate and has an algorithm that switches the dose setting to a higher dose with a higher respiratory rate. As the patient breathes faster the dose will increase; as the patient breathes slower, the dose will return to a lower setting. This technique allows the patient to increase the dose of oxygen with demand without manually changing the dose setting.

Oximeter regulated flow: This type of OCD device monitors the patient's oxygen saturation. An algorithm in the device changes the oxygen dose based on oxygen saturation. There is an approved product with this feature, but it is not commercially available at the present time.

Motion regulated flow: This device senses movement and changes the oxygen dose to a higher setting. When movement stops, the OCD then switches back to the lower dose setting. There is an approved product on the market.

Patient delivery interface devices

Nasal cannula has been the standard for low flow oxygen delivery. The cannula options have included multiple lengths for specific applications, different materials (plastic, silicone, etc.), different diameter nasal prong lumen, and accessories for comfort. Lumen size and tubing length have an impact on oxygen delivery, and if the cannula is changed to a different capability, the flow and patient oximetry should be checked. Single lumen cannulas are typical and account for a majority of cannula options. Dual lumen cannula are used with demand flow conserving devices.

Other interface devices include:

Nasal mask: If the nasal cannula prongs are causing irritation, the nasal mask can be used as an option. The nasal mask cups oxygen around the nose to eliminate the prongs entering the nose. The nasal mask must be used with continuous flow oxygen, as the conserving type systems would not be able to sense an inspiration and function properly.

Headset oxygen: Headset low flow oxygen delivery was originally designed to provide a solution for people who felt the cannula put too much pressure on the ears and cheeks. Headsets are used with prolonged phone use, so this appeared to be a good option for patients using home oxygen.

Oxygen glasses: Oxygen glasses have the same potential advantages as the headset. The oxygen glasses also add an esthetic value, as many people cannot tell that a patient is wearing oxygen at all. The author of this book was known to wear the oxygen glasses at a major conference without being recognized as a LTOT patient.

Transtracheal oxygen: Transtracheal oxygen delivery is described in another chapter of this book. *(See Chapter 7)*

Oxygen delivery accessory items

There are also many accessories to help make oxygen use easier to handle:

Carts: Carts have helped patients be more mobile with their oxygen systems. Originally, oxygen carts were the same as those used in the hospital. Lightweight functional carts are now available for the home oxygen patient's use.

Backpacks: Backpacks became a request of patients who wanted to have more free use of their hands. A user friendly backpack allows for more mobility during activities of daily living than is typically possible with a shoulder strap.

Shoulder straps: Shoulder straps have evolved to more comfortable, aesthetically pleasing options. Some shoulder straps are made of elastic material that can act as a shock absorber for the pressure transferred to the shoulder.

Liter meters: Liter meters are used to spot check the continuous flow from a low flow oxygen device. These devices are used by home care providers to check accuracy of the flow setting, yet patients can do the same spot check with proper training and availability of the tool.

Pulse meters: A pulse meter is a device that checks the pulse volume of a pulse style intermittent flow device. This product is used by home care providers. It is more expensive than a liter meter.

Batteries: Batteries are an option for POCs, as the operation time away from an AC or DC source is determined by the use time of the battery. Additional fully charged batteries can extend use time and are an important factor for air travel. Pulse style conserving devices have a set battery life, so extra batteries should be available for the system as back up.

Oximeters: Oximeters have become a more common tool used by oxygen patients. Initial concern from clinicians regarding a patient's use of personal oximeters has been reduced as they have recognized the benefits of proper oxygen settings for different activity levels, and patients have received improved education on the use of these devices. As Dr. Petty recommended, patients should "Titrate as You Migrate."

Home oxygen delivery options

The oxygen provider delivers oxygen. This was the standard of care until recent payment cuts forced home care providers to search for other options. In the past, providers offered services and equipment for the home oxygen patient. The patient did not need to be concerned with products or services, as this was all covered by the provider. Now payers have decided that they only want to pay for equipment, so the services that have been offered in the past may be changing. Home oxygen patients need to be informed of their options and stay actively involved in their home oxygen program.

Non-delivery for stationary oxygen or portables has emerged as a method of providing LTOT in the home. This method provides for a home oxygen system that does not require frequent deliveries from the provider. With this method the provider may not see the patient as frequently, so the patient needs to be proactive to identify problems and communicate with the provider for any oxygen needs.

Patients obtaining refills from the provider has been considered inappropriate in the past, yet if the patient has the ability and desire to pick up his oxygen refills from a provider, it gives the patient more control of portable oxygen refills and can assist the oxygen provider. This would be similar to the patient picking up other medicine refills from a local pharmacy. Again, the market is changing and new methods are being considered.

Commercial carriers delivering oxygen to the patient's home has been considered. The Post Office or UPS could make routine deliveries to the home. The issue with commercial carriers is that they are not medically trained. Patients need to make sure they have proper instruction on use, application, and safety from the provider or responsible clinicians if a commercial delivery of oxygen is utilized.

Key issues in oxygen therapy

Proper oxygen saturation: One primary objective of LTOT is to ensure that the oxygen delivered to the patient reaches gas exchange units (alveoli) in the lung. Oxygen delivered anytime during the breathing cycle that does not reach a gas exchange unit is considered wasted. The goal for efficient oxygen delivery is the proper percent of oxygen saturation or oxygen pressure (PAO_2) in the blood at all activity levels. It is important to note that oxygen savings is considered accomplished only after the patient is adequately oxygenated and is a secondary objective for device performance.

Ventilation and perfusion issues: A patient's respiratory physiology is a very dynamic process. Even if an oxygen device is providing consistent oxygen delivery, results can vary for an individual patient from moment to moment, and also between groups of patients using similar devices. This issue, combined with the wide variety of performance differences of oxygen systems, has created a very difficult challenge for clinicians and patients to maintain proper oxygenation.

Activity levels: Several variables may affect a patient's oxygenation while using an oxygen delivery system. Increased respiratory rate will shorten inspiratory time and may reduce the amount of oxygen a patient will receive. In the past, an exercise prescription was written for patients whose increase in respiratory rate with exercise required more oxygen to maintain proper saturation levels. This increase in flow rate was to compensate for a shorter inspiratory time due to the faster respiratory rate. The general rule of thumb was to double the patient's flow rate (e.g. from 2 lpm to 4 lpm) during exercise. **Oxygen dependent patients should always be tested on their oxygen system at different activity levels — sleep, rest, and exercise, as well as at altitude — to ensure the device meets their oxygenation needs at all levels of activity.** Any change in respiratory rate or pattern may affect the patient's oxygenation. The lack of attention to this variable in the past has created the misperception that conserving devices do not oxygenate effectively.

Titration: A titration test is the standard method of measuring patients' oxygen needs with exercise. It is a simple method that only requires an oximeter and a place to exercise. If a patient will be doing more strenuous activity, every attempt should be made to simulate that activity to see if the device properly oxygenates the user. Sleeping with an OCD is possible, yet an overnight oximetry test is strongly recommended to determine if the device is triggering with each breath and maintaining patient oxygen saturation.

Altitude: Altitude has an impact on the pressure of oxygen, not necessarily the amount of oxygen. Oxygen devices will give approximately the same volume of oxygen at higher altitudes (or in an airplane), but the pressure differences at different altitudes may have an impact on oxygenation levels. It is important to understand that if an oxygen system is able to meet a patient's oxygen needs at a lower altitude, it is possible that that same system may not be able to meet the patient's needs at a higher altitude. Unfortunately, it is generally not feasible to test patients on their oxygen systems at pressures that they would be experiencing at varying altitudes. In general, the common practice has been to double the device's delivery setting when the patient is at altitude. However, if the oxygen system the patient is using is already running at its top setting at a lower altitude, another system should be considered for use at higher altitudes. This is where a personal oximeter is of great benefit.

Equivalency: When OCDs first entered the LTOT market, they were revolutionary, not evolutionary. A revolutionary product has no predecessor; therefore, there is nothing to compare the product with. For OCD manufacturers to be able to enter the market and sell their products, OCDs needed a reference point that could be understood by the persons using the device. Continuous flow oxygen (CFO) delivery was the gold standard in oxygen therapy up to this point, so an attempt was made to compare the effectiveness and delivery of the OCD to the CFO gold standard. Intermittent flow devices such as OCDs deliver a certain volume of gas with each sensed patient breath. A patient breathing on a CFO device receives a variable volume of gas dependent on their breathing profile. By selecting one breathing pattern and one breath rate, a delivered dose volume of oxygen can be made equivalent to the volume taken in during continuous flow of oxygen. As a result, manufacturers selected a volume of oxygen for a given device setting that they felt would be equivalent to continuous flow and made that the flow setting on their device. However, this concept only works if the patient never changes his breathing pattern. Obviously, that is not the case in real life. A setting of 1 to 3 liters on an OCD might better be shown as A, B, and C, as this could be less confusing to patients. Patients often believe that the 1 or 3 designation is equivalent to 1 or 3 liters.

Graph: Oxygenation in test lung study of seven oxygen conserving devices all set on "2".

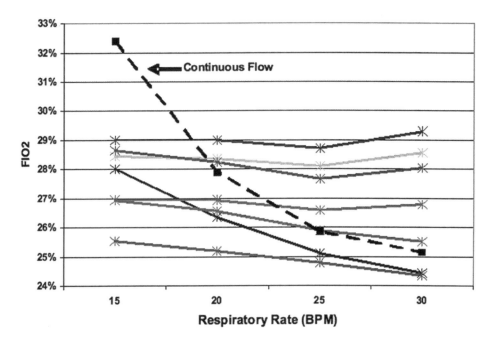

Most OCDs have a number on the selector dial and, even though they claim to deliver oxygen equivalently to continuous flow at that same setting, typically are not equivalent to CFO, let alone any other conserving device at that setting. The graph shown here displays the delivered FIO_2 values for seven conserving devices, all of which are set at the device setting of 2. As can be seen, there is a wide variety in delivered FIO_2, and no device could be considered to have delivered therapy equivalent to CFO.

Standards for OCDs: There are few standards for the development of OCDs. This lack of standards has led to a wide variety in device performance and has fostered confusion in the market. Using the scenario outlined above as an example, the setting numbers on the dials do not relate to any manufacturing standard and were generally meant to be used only as a comparison to continuous flow. As shown above, this is not a viable comparison. So this begs the question, "What does '2' really stand for?" With minimal standards regulating the manufacture of OCDs, the answer must be this:

The 2 does not mean "liters per minute" or signify a specific volume of oxygen. In fact, it doesn't mean much of anything. It is only a reference point to be used to test the patient and to turn the selector, if necessary, to obtain the proper oxygen saturation in the patient. (An easy analogy for this situation would be if you just saw the number 50 on a speedometer. Is that kilometers per hour? Miles per minute? Furlongs per day? That kind of information would be nice to know if you find yourself in a speed trap!)

Savings ratio: Oxygen saving is possible with conserving devices; therefore a ratio of oxygen use by an OCD compared to oxygen use by CFO therapy can be calculated. One can increase this savings ratio by decreasing the oxygen delivery by the device. This has been the basis for many manufacturers' claims of high oxygen savings.

Dose volume: The dose volume from an OCD determines the FIO2 by the patient. A higher dose volume generally means a higher FIO2 at a constant, normal breathing volume (tidal volume). Dose volumes from various OCDs are different at the same numerical setting. Prior to using any OCD, the dose volume per setting should be determined. Some devices have limited maximum dose volumes and, as a result, are not suitable for patients requiring higher FIO2 at certain activity levels.

Triggering sensitivity: The triggering sensitivity determines if and/or when a conserving device will deliver a volume of oxygen. All conserving devices need to sense a patient's inhalation to initiate the flow of oxygen. Some devices are more sensitive than others, meaning those devices will trigger their oxygen flow sooner than the others. The first half of inspiration is important in oxygen delivery — if a conserving device is slow to respond to an inspiratory signal, it may deliver oxygen late in the inspiratory cycle and the delivered oxygen may not go to gas exchange units in the lung. Additionally, if the device does not sense a breath at all, it will not deliver its dose volume, and the patient will not receive oxygen for that breath. At activity, most patients have a strong signal, and most devices will trigger without issue. However, sleeping patients may not generate much of an inspiratory signal and oxygen delivery may be missed on weak breaths. It is recommended that a patient wishing to use their conserving device during sleep undergo an overnight oximetry study with the device prior to using it in the home. If the device does not sense a breath, the patient will not receive oxygen for that breath.

Timing of oxygen delivery: There is an undefined "sweet spot" where oxygen delivery is most effective. Any oxygen delivery outside that sweet spot is wasted and does not provide oxygen to the patient's gas exchange units. Typically, oxygen delivered in the first half of inspiration goes to the alveoli, the gas exchange units in the lung. Oxygen delivered after a certain point in the second half of inspiration remains in the conductive passages in the lung, where no gas exchange occurs, and is eventually exhaled. Most pulse delivery style conserving devices attempt to deliver their entire oxygen dose within the first half of inspiration. Demand and hybrid conserving devices, by design, deliver oxygen all the way to the end of the inspiratory cycle, only turning off when the patient exhales. This means that the oxygen delivered near the end of inhalation is generally wasted, but the patient still receives the majority of the delivered volume.

Cannula: single lumen vs. dual lumen; nasal prong style: Most pneumatic conserving devices require use of a dual lumen cannula — one lumen to sense the breath and the other lumen to deliver the oxygen. Some pneumatic devices use a single lumen and thus have a unique way of ending oxygen delivery. Electronic devices only need a single lumen cannula since a circuit times the end of the delivery. The size and shape of the cannula nasal prongs is also an issue to be aware of when using OCDs. Some cannula feature flared tips, some straight tips, and others tapered tips. These design differences alter the resistance to flow inside the cannula, which can affect the amount of oxygen being delivered to the patient. Pediatric or low flow cannulas are not recommended for most conserving devices as the resistance to flow can impact the triggering of the device and can cause the conserver to auto cycle. Note that dual lumen cannula cannot be used with transtracheal oxygen delivery.

Cylinder operating pressure: OCDs utilizing oxygen cylinders are usually rated for a specific cylinder operating pressure, often from 500 psi to 2000 psi. It is important that the OCD be switched to a compatible tank when the current tank pressure is outside of the specified pressure range for operation. Also, many pneumatic conserver delivery volumes change with a change in tank pressure. Some devices will deliver slightly lower dose volumes at 500 psi than they will at 2000 psi. These volumes are usually not significant, but should be noted. Devices with continuous flow capability will see delivered flow rates drop as the cylinder pressure drops.

Ease of use: Extra features and benefits are often not utilized by patients using conserving devices. Adding clinical features are only an advantage if the patient's clinician sets the device up and knows how and why a special feature is a benefit to the patient. The "keep it simple" philosophy is an advantage for patients and helps keep confusion with a device to a minimum. A few devices released in the last few years have additional features unique to that device.

Other application issues:

- OCDs should never be used with in-line humidifiers as the OCD will not be properly triggered.

- Long delivery tubing will slow the gas delivery and may affect device sensitivity. Refer to individual manufacturer recommendations before using non-standard lengths of tubing, and always test the patient's saturation when using longer delivery tubing.

- OCDs should not be used with a mask as the OCD will not sense an inspiratory signal and there is no oxygen delivery during exhalation to flush the resulting deadspace volume.

- OCDs should not be used to bleed in oxygen to a CPAP or Bi-Level device as the system will not properly trigger and oxygen flow/volume will not be adequate to change FIO2.

Oxygen delivery fundamentals

To adequately understand OCDs, it is first beneficial to think about continuous flow oxygen delivery, which, for decades was considered the "gold standard" of LTOT. As CFO is applied via nasal cannula, some of the oxygen delivered during inhalation is mixed with inspired air for a net FIO_2 in the lungs. Unfortunately, determining FIO_2 isn't quite as simple as calculating the flow of oxygen and the flow of air. Several factors conspire to complicate the process:

Dilution: During CFO the flow rate is fixed, so as a patient breathes faster, creating a shorter inhalation time, the amount of oxygen inhaled per breath decreases. As a result, the net FIO2 drops.

Dead space: During the latter portion of inhalation, gas entering the airway never reaches the lungs, but remains in the connecting air passages ("plumbing") leading to gas exchange units only to be exhaled. This includes some of the CFO, which is, of course, wasted. The amount varies with the patient's anatomy and breathing pattern.

Pooling: On the other hand, oxygen delivered late in exhalation, when the patient's expiratory flow rate is relatively low, or during the pause after total exhalation, may not be wasted. The oxygen exiting the small diameter cannula is traveling at a relatively high velocity, and some amount of oxygen is "pooled" in and around the nose, nasopharynx, and upper airway. This oxygen is able to be inspired at the beginning of inhalation. Patient disease, anatomy, and breathing pattern, as well as environmental conditions (like wind), can vary this effect.

The chart on this page highlights these factors, and indicates what is considered to be "useful" oxygen during continuous flow therapy.

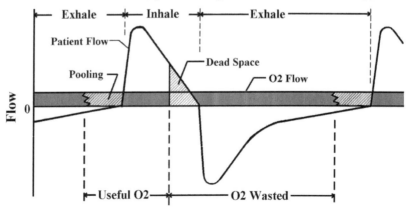

Gerald Durkan, whose product development work led to the products and patents now marketed by Sunrise Medical, thought that it would be advantageous to deliver the same 33 mL dose from 2 lpm continuous flow oxygen therapy early in inhalation, but at a higher flow rate and for a much shorter duration. *(See following graph.)* With this method of delivery, the delivered pulse volume could easily be changed by varying the duration of the delivery. Most, but not all, pulse devices today operate in this manner, increasing the delivery time with an increase in the setting number.

Graph: Early Conserving Concepts: Intermittent Oxygen Delivery via Pulse Delivery Device

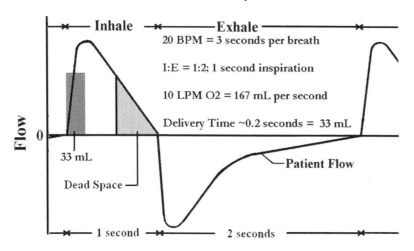

Making an informed decision

The use of long term oxygen therapy continues to grow. There is no one right product for all applications of oxygen therapy. The patient's needs are the driving factor, and it is important to understand that every person's needs will be very different. Understanding the capabilities of all oxygen therapy equipment on the market will give users, clinicians, marketers, and manufacturers knowledge that can be used to ask the right questions, evaluate the user's needs, and make an informed decision when buying and using oxygen.

"May the holes in your net be no larger than the fish in it."
Irish Blessing

Chapter 20

Current Research in Long-Term Oxygen Therapy

Richard Casaburi, PhD, MD

More than 40 years ago, Tom Petty and his colleagues established that long-term oxygen therapy radically improved the prognosis of people whose oxygen levels were low when they were at rest. This seminal study spurred the creation of a large industry whose goal is to provide oxygen therapy to those who need it. In the United States today, more than a million patients receive long-term oxygen therapy. A large fraction of these patients carry the diagnosis of chronic obstructive pulmonary disease (COPD). The annual cost of long-term oxygen therapy in the United States is said to exceed three billion dollars.

Interestingly, the per capita use of long-term oxygen therapy is several-fold greater in the United States than in any other country in the world. This difference is too large to be explained by difference in disease patterns among countries. It also cannot be explained by lack of access. Many countries, especially those in Europe and East Asia, have well-developed systems for providing oxygen therapy. These differences seem more likely to be related to differing prescribing practices and differing adherence to prescribing guidelines. They also relate to the way in which patient's oxygen needs are followed.

In seeking the source of these differences, it is instructive to consider the guidelines we follow in using oxygen supplementation for three specific situations: during exercise, during air flight and during sleep. We can consider whether the guidelines we follow are evidence based and discuss the specific benefits we expect to reap when we give supplemental oxygen.

Do we, in the United States, give long-term oxygen therapy to too many or too few patients?

Should many more COPD patients receive oxygen during exercise, air flight and sleep?

Exercise: The argument for providing a wider range of patients with supplemental oxygen during exercise seems quite easy to make. It is crystal clear that supplemental oxygen improves exercise tolerance in patients with COPD. Physiological studies have shown, that, at a given level of exercise, supplemental oxygen decreases shortness of breath, decreases the level of pulmonary ventilation and decreases dynamic hyperinflation. The blood vessels in the lung also dilate allowing pulmonary artery pressure to decrease. Studies in our laboratory have shown that this occurs even in COPD patients whose oxygen levels are generally felt to be high enough to not require oxygen supplementation (above an arterial oxygen saturation of 88%). We were able to show that providing supplemental oxygen to a group of COPD patients whose oxygen saturation during exercise averaged 92% yielded substantially less dyspnea and resulted in lower levels of pulmonary ventilation at a given level of exercise. The amount of time that these subjects were able to tolerate a given exercise work rate more than doubled.

A further argument in favor of providing more patients with oxygen during exercise is that technologic advances have made ambulatory oxygen therapy more practical. The time is long past when ambulatory oxygen meant a heavy compressed gas tank mounted in a cart designed to be dragged behind the patient. Ten years ago, Tom Petty and the other members of the 5th Oxygen Consensus Conference enunciated the principle that ambulatory oxygen should be *defined* as a device weighing 10 lbs. or less. Today, we have met and well exceeded this goal: each of the modalities listed below are available in configurations weighing less than 5 lbs.

- Lightweight, small compressed gas cylinders, capable of high filling pressures are readily available.
- Liquid oxygen stores the most oxygen in a given volume; compact units with easy refilling capabilities are commonly in use.
- Battery-powered portable oxygen concentrators are a high-technology solution to ambulatory needs. Importantly, these devices do not require home oxygen delivery.

These arguments suggest that we should be providing supplemental oxygen during ambulatory activities of daily living to a wider range of patients.

Air Flight: Commercial air flights are pressurized to a pressure equivalent to an altitude of 8000 ft.; this has the same effect as breathing 15% oxygen at sea level. Clearly, those who require supplemental oxygen at sea level will have to use it during air flight, but how many others who otherwise do not require oxygen at sea level need it during air flight? This is important, because obtaining supplemental oxygen for air flight is a rather inconvenient and expensive endeavor. Typical recommendations allow that COPD patients whose arterial oxygen partial pressure is greater than 70 mmHg at sea level are OK to fly without any further evaluation. Those with lower arterial oxygen partial pressures are recommended to undergo an altitude simulation test and, if low oxygen levels are seen, use supplemental oxygen during air flight. But these guidelines have been questioned. It has been shown that a substantial fraction of COPD patients whose oxygen levels are in the normal range at sea level nonetheless will experience oxygen levels during air flight that are low enough to meet guidelines for oxygen supplementation…especially when the patient performs a bit of activity that might be encountered walking in the airplane aisles.

These considerations would argue that a wider range of COPD patients should be tested for their need for supplemental oxygen when they fly.

Sleep: It is generally recommended that those COPD patients who experience low levels of oxygen in their arterial blood while sleeping be given supplemental oxygen when they sleep even if their oxygen levels when they are awake are satisfactory. Studies have shown that a substantial fraction (perhaps 25%) of severe COPD patients fall into this category. It can be argued that overnight oximetry, a test capable of detecting low oxygen levels during sleep, should be performed widely in COPD patients. Implementing this screening would clearly result in a larger number of COPD patients receiving nocturnal oxygen.

Should many fewer COPD patients receive oxygen during exercise, air flight, and sleep?

This argument needs to be framed by considering the underlying reason for prescribing supplemental oxygen. Is it to keep arterial oxygen levels above some limit? This can't be the correct answer, since these limits are empiric and not firmly tied to patient-centered outcomes. Is it to improve symptoms? This might be entertained. After all, supplemental oxygen decreases shortness of breath, enhances exercise capacity and improves cognition (among other benefits). But would a therapy that yielded purely symptomatic benefits be readily embraced despite a price tag of roughly $3 billion annually? No, the primary reason that we prescribe long-term oxygen therapy is that it substantially improves prognosis in COPD by slowing disease progression and decreasing mortality.

Can an argument be made that oxygen supplementation improves prognosis in COPD patients who experience low oxygen levels during exercise, air flight, and sleep?

Exercise: It can be succinctly stated that no study has shown better long-term outcomes are achieved when patients are given ambulatory oxygen during exercise. This applies to patients whose oxygen levels are low only during exertion. Surprisingly, it also applies to patients whose oxygen levels are low both during rest and during exertion. It is entirely possible that providing oxygen solely at rest would yield the impressive mortality benefits that Tom Petty and his colleagues observed.

Moreover, it may be questioned whether the pattern of usage seen in most patients who receive ambulatory oxygen is likely to produce an improved prognosis. One of the messages that came out of the NOTT study (headed by Tom Petty, performed in the United States) and the MRC trial (headed by David Flenley, performed in Great Britain) was that improvements in mortality correlated with the number of hours per day that hypoxemia was treated. Recent studies suggest that those who are prescribed ambulatory oxygen generally use it for only a small number of hours daily. It seems quite plausible that avoiding only a few hours of low oxygen levels a day will not affect long-term prognosis.

Providing ambulatory oxygen therapy is quite expensive – considerably more expensive than providing stationary oxygen. Should we limit its use in view of lack of evidence of long-term benefit?

Air Flight: Here the argument regarding long-term benefits is even clearer. It is hard to postulate that avoiding the few hours of low oxygen levels that the occasional flier might experience during an air flight would influence their long-term prognosis. (An exception might be those patients with concomitant cardiac disease in whom low oxygen levels might trigger acute problems). Indeed, in studies of altitude simulation, few patients complain of appreciable symptoms when their oxygen levels fall, much less long-term sequelae. Should recommendations of oxygen during air flight be limited to the more frail COPD patient who might be more likely to suffer acutely from its lack?

Sleep: A single study can be cited that demonstrates a long-term benefit when patients with low oxygen levels (only low during sleep) were treated with nighttime oxygen. The study of Fletcher and his colleagues showed that pulmonary artery pressure elevations were decreased when patients with nighttime low oxygen levels were treated with nighttime oxygen therapy, certainly a beneficial effect. Yet in Fletcher's study no improvement in survival was detected. A more recent study from France similarly was unable to detect a survival advantage resulting from nocturnal oxygen therapy. Should nocturnal oxygen therapy be limited to those with co-morbidities (e.g., cardiac disease, right heart failure) that suggest elevated risk of harm from low oxygen levels?

How can these opposing points of view be resolved? No amount of theoretical argument will suffice. The obvious answer is that clinical research studies are necessary to demonstrate whether oxygen therapy during exercise, air flight, and sleep affects long-term prognosis of COPD patients. Why haven't these studies been performed already? Two parties with deep pockets have a strong interest in establishing the indications for long-term oxygen therapy. Oxygen suppliers and equipment manufacturers have shown little willingness to fund research to evaluate the indications for their "product." This is in marked contrast with the pharmaceutical industry, whose budget for research and development of drugs is substantial. It might be argued that the oxygen industry is different in that each supplier and manufacturer deals with the same "product" (oxygen), whereas the pharmaceutical industry funds research into their own proprietary drug. Yet many examples can be found where the pharmaceutical industry funds projects that yield broad benefits that go well beyond single drug products.

The second party with strong interest in these questions is the group of payers that fund oxygen therapy. Though insurers play a part, the substantial majority of people who receive long-term oxygen therapy in the

United States are Medicare or Medicaid beneficiaries. So it is the Federal government who is the major payer. Yet, until recently, research into oxygen therapy received little attention. A seminal event was the convening of a workshop by the National Heart Lung and Blood Institute (a branch of the National Institutes of Health) in 2004; the purpose of this meeting was to establish priorities for research into long-term oxygen therapy. A workshop report was published in early 2006.1 This report laid out the current state of knowledge and prioritized studies to answer the important questions.

It can be argued that there are four key trials that are needed to establish rational prescribing practices for long-term oxygen therapy:

1) Stationary oxygen + ambulatory oxygen vs. stationary oxygen alone for patients who have low oxygen levels both at rest and during exercise

2) Ambulatory oxygen vs. no oxygen for patients who have normal oxygen levels at rest and low oxygen levels with exercise

3) Night-time oxygen vs. no oxygen for patients who have normal oxygen levels at rest and low oxygen levels with sleep

4) Stationary oxygen + ambulatory oxygen vs. no oxygen for patients with mildly low oxygen levels at rest

In considering how to conduct these individual studies a few principles of design are similar, regardless of which question is addressed. First, these need to be randomized trials, with recruited participants agreeing to be assigned to either of the two study groups. Second, the primary outcome should be mortality; such trials need several years to have a chance of determining a difference in survival. Third, these trials need to incorporate a large study group.*

Studies as large as these are expensive to organize and require a large number of research centers to participate. Consider also that these trials also have considerable logistical difficulties. The most daunting is the need to assure that volunteers who agree to participate in the protocol actually adhere to the assigned therapy. For example, consider participants in the fourth trial described above who are assigned to the oxygen therapy group. These subjects cannot be told that adhering to the instructions to utilize supplemental oxygen full-time will be of benefit to them (because it is unknown whether there will be any benefit), only that it will be beneficial to the *trial* that they adhere. How many subjects will faithfully adhere to this intrusive and inconvenient therapy over a period of several years? Clearly, if adherence is poor, the study will fail to test its hypothesis.

A study of the kind described has been taken on by the National Heart Lung and Blood Institute (with the assistance of the Center for Medicare and Medicaid Services). Fourteen regional centers around the country have been identified and charged with designing the study and recruiting the subjects. The study is in the early stages of subject recruitment. Please wish us luck with this endeavor!

"Calling fishing a hobby is like calling brain surgery a job."
— Paul Schullery—

RESOURCES

Throughout this book there are many references to helpful web site links. Those, as well as a few additional ones, are listed here:

American Association for Respiratory Care	www.aarc.org
American Cancer Society	www.cancer.org
American Lung Association	www.lungusa.org
American Thoracic Society	www.thoracic.org
Ask Dr. Tom	www.yourlunghealth.org
Aspen Lung Conference	www.uchsc.edu/pulmonary/aspen
Chest Foundation of the American College of Chest Physicians	www.chestfoundation.org/ foundation/petty.php
Colorado COPD Connection	www.copdconnectco.org
COPD Alert	www.copd-alert.com
COPD Canada Patient Network	www.copdcanada.ca
COPD Digest	www.copddigest.org
COPD Foundation	research.copdfoundation.org/
COPD Guide	www.copdguide.com/?WT. srch=1&sc=SPRACQWEB SEMGOG1001020
COPDGene	www.copdgene.org/
Dr. Tom Petty	www.drtompetty.org
Emphysema Foundation for Our Right to Survive (EFFORTS)	www.emphysema.net
Everything Respiratory Magazine	www.ERmag.org
Frontline Advice for COPD Patients co-edited by Drs. Tom Petty & Jim Good	www.drtompetty.org www.nlhep.org/resources.html

GOLD (Global Initiative for Chronic Obstructive Lung Disease)	www.goldcopd.org
LTOT Network	www.ltotnet.org/resources.html
Lyn Cole's Blog	profiles.yahoo.com/u/KIEVF7SMP EV62PAF7LWHN3HEWU
National Emphysema Foundation (Dr. Sree Nair)	www.emphysemafoundation.org
National Heart Lung and Blood Institute	www.nhlbi.nih.gov/health/ public/lung/copd/
National Home Oxygen Patient Association	www.homeoxygen.org/member.html
National Lung Health Education Program (NLHEP)	www.nlhep.org
Nonin Oximeter Booklet written by Dr. Petty	www.nonin.com/documents/go2/ 6965-00001%20Dr%20Petty %20GO2%20Brochure_ENG.pdf
Pulmonary Education & Research Foundation	www.perf2ndwind.org/
Pulmonary Education & Research Foundation (PERF) Letters From Tom "Titrate When You Migrate"	www.perf2ndwind.org/html/tom petty/2006/Nov-2006.html
SCOOP Transtracheal Oxygen Therapy	www.tto2.com
Soft Hose Cannulas	www.softhose.com
Summaries of the Six Oxygen Consensus Conferences	www.ltotnet.org/resources.html
The Pulmonary Paper	www.pulmonarypaper.org/
World Health Organization	www.who.int

GLOSSARY

Alveoli	The final branchings of the respiratory tree
Arterial carbon dioxide	Carbon dioxide in arterial blood (PaCO 2)
Blood gas analysis (ABG)	Also called arterial blood gas (ABG), is a test which measures the amounts of oxygen and carbon dioxide in the blood, as well as the acidity (pH) of the blood.
British Medical Research Council (MRC)	British Medical Research Council sponsored first major LTOT study in Britain
Bronchiolitis obliterans	Inflammatory damage and obstruction of the small airways of the lungs
Carbon monoxide measurements	A colorless, odorless, poisonous gas measurement
Carboxyhemoglobin	Carbon monoxide mixes and binds with hemoglobin in the blood to form carboxyhemoglobin (COHb). The process of carbon monoxide binding to hemoglobin reduces the amount of oxygen being transported to body tissues and vital organs such as the brain and heart.
Chest radiography	Chest x-ray
Chronic bronchitis	A chronic inflammation of the bronchi (medium-size airways) in the lungs
CO_2	Carbon dioxide
Cor pulmonale	Failure of the right side of the heart brought on by long-term high blood pressure in the pulmonary arteries and right ventricle of the heart
CPAP	Continuous Positive Airway Pressure is an effective treatment for Sleep Apnea patients
Cryocooler	A cryocooler chills gas into a liquid form. The Dewar is what the liquid oxygen is stored in.
Diffusion	Diffusion capacity is a measurement of the lung's ability to transfer gases
Dyspnea	Shortness of breath; labored or difficult breathing
EKG	Electrocardiogram
Electrocardiogram (ECG or EKG)	A test that records the electrical activity of or history of specific heart diseases or other medical conditions
Exacerbation	An increase in the severity of a disease or in any of its signs or symptoms
Fulminating	Rapid, sudden, and severe such as an infection, fever, or hemorrhage
Lung function test (FEV_1)	Forced Expiratory Volume in one second

Hematocrit	A blood test that measures the percentage of red blood cells found in whole blood
Humidifier	A household appliance that increases humidity (moisture) in a single room or in the entire home
Hypoxemia	Decreased partial pressure of oxygen in blood; sometimes specifically as less than 60 mmHg (8.0 kPa)
Hypoxemic	Abnormal condition resulting from a decrease in the oxygen supplied to or utilized by body tissue
ILD	Interstitial lung disease
LTOT	Long term oxygen therapy
LVRS	Lung volume reduction surgery
Nasal cannulae	A device used to deliver supplemental oxygen to a patient. This device consists of a plastic tube which fits behind the ears, and a set of two prongs which are placed in the nostrils.
Nocturnal pulmonary edema	An accumulation of an excessive amount of watery fluid in the lungs
NOTT	Nocturnal Oxygen Therapy Trial
OCD	Oxygen conserving device
OSA	Obstructive sleep apnea
Oxygen Saturation	Percent of oxygen in the blood
Palliation	To relieve or lessen a disease without curing
PaO2	Oxygen partial pressure in arterial blood
PFT	Pulmonary function test
Polycythemia	An increase above the normal in the number of red cells in the blood
Pulmonary fibrosis	Formation or development of excess fibrous connective tissue in the lungs; sometimes described as scarring of the lungs
Pulmonary hypertension	High blood pressure in the arteries that supply the lungs
Pulse oximetry	A non-invasive method for monitoring the oxygenation of a patients blood.
Right ventricle hypertrophy	A form of ventricular hypertrophy affecting the right ventricle; blood travels through the right ventricle to the lungs
Spirometry or Spirography	Pulmonary function test (PFT) that is a graphic measurement of breathing, including breathing movements and breathing capacity
Stent	A man-made 'tube' inserted into a natural passage/conduit in the body to prevent, or counteract, a disease-induced, localized flow constriction
TB sequelae	Defined as the state with various secondary complications after healing of TB, such as chronic respiratory failure (CRF), cor pulmonale or chronic pulmonary inflammation
Titrate	Measure
Tonometric	Any of various instruments for measuring pressure or tension

"The gods do not deduct from man's allotted span the hours spent in fishing."
— Babylonian Proverb —

Biographies

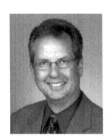

Robert McCoy BS RRT FAARC is the managing director of Valley Inspired Products Inc. (VIP) www.inspire-drc.com a research and testing company located in Apple Valley MN. He also manages ValleyAire Home Respiratory Services Inc. a HME provider of respiratory products and services. Both companies conduct research on products and services with VIP doing bench studies and ValleyAire conducting field studies. Bob has worked in all segments of oxygen therapy starting out as a staff RT in a hospital and progressing to Director of a large respiratory department. Moving to industry, Bob has been a product manager, marketing manager, and finally a Director of Marketing for a large respiratory manufacturer before starting VIP.

Bob is active in his professional organization with an appointment by the AARC to represent the organization to ASTM (which develops international standards for materials, products, systems and services used in construction, manufacturing and transportation) and has been elected to the chairman position of the home care section of the AARC. Bob has published peer review articles in professional journals, written for trade magazines, lectured at both state and national meetings and has participated in numerous LTOT consensus conferences. Known as a patient advocate, Bob can quite often be found meeting with an oxygen patient to discuss challenges the patients have and what needs to be addressed to meet the patient's needs.

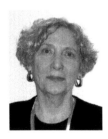

Louise M. Nett, RN, RRT, FAARC started her career in the respiratory field in 1965 working with Dr. Thomas Petty. At that time Respiratory Care was in it's infancy. Louise and Tom developed the Respiratory Intensive Care unit at the University of Colorado. Soon after they realized that many of their patients were readmitted for the same diagnosis. The need for rehabilitation was obvious. They were funded by a government grant to study this new field of pulmonary rehabilitation and LTOT. Then followed many conferences in Denver, the US, and many foreign countries teaching the principles learned from the grant. In later years she focused her attention on the role of the RT and RN on Smoking Cessation. Louise and Tom teamed on lots of respiratory projects, conferences, articles and books. This book was in development when Dr. Petty died Dec.12, 2009. Kay Bowen and Louise took on the responsibility for bringing the book to completion starting on Jan 2, 2010. Louise has been a dedicated professional for 51 years but finds time for other interests....fishing, hunting, and watercolor and acrylic painting.

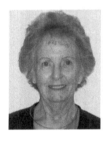

Kay Bowen first heard the name Dr. Tom Petty in the early 1960s when her father, who lived in rural Eastern Colorado, was referred to Dr. Petty and diagnosed with emphysema. Many years later, working as a secretary in Continuing Medical Education at Presbyterian Hospital, she learned that Dr. Petty would soon become the new Director of Academic Affairs at Presbyterian Hospital. Shortly thereafter Kay successfully interviewed for a job as his manuscript secretary. Of course, she knew that Dr. Petty was adamantly opposed to smoking, so it was on January 1, 1989, that she gave up smoking and began her new job working for Dr. Petty. Kay enjoyed her work and was honored to have a small part in his many articles and books written over the last 20 years. Most challenging projects would include the *Year Books of Pulmonary Diseases* and *The History of the Aspen Lung Conference.* With the completion of *Adventures of an Oxy-Phile$_2$*, Kay will spend more time gardening and quilting.

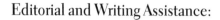

Editorial and Writing Assistance:

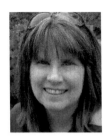

Debbie Bunch, BA (Editor and Writer) is a long time writer for the American Association for Respiratory Care and it's magazine, *AARC Times*. Over the years she had many opportunities to interview Dr. Tom Petty for stories of interest to the respiratory therapy profession and always found him to be most willing to share his expertise with her readers. In 2003 she had the distinct honor of interviewing Dr. Petty about his life's work for the *AARC Times* article "Just Call Him 'Doc,'" which ran in the October issue and commemorated his receipt of the 2003 Jimmy A. Young Medal, the AARC's highest honor.

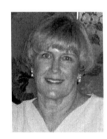

Diane Seebass, BA, MA (Assistant Editor) is the "bean counter" of the editing world, doing mostly copyediting (dotting I's and crossing t's, checking grammar and mechanics) and adding a little developmental work when I see the need. After attending DePauw University and the University of Colorado, I earned a teaching degree in English and French from Colorado State College. Later, after teaching high school senior English, I took a master's degree in Modern Letters at the University of Tulsa. When I met Dr. Petty, I was teaching composition at Tulsa Community College, doing some freelance work, and doing fiction editing for the *Nimrod International Journal*. It has been my pleasure to work on his manuscripts and learn more about his subject matter, usually pulmonary medicine, while enjoying his acute sense of humor. A few of his interesting books became *Pulmonary Diseases of the Elderly* in 2007, the *History of the Thomas L. Petty Aspen Lung Conference*, and *From Both Ends of the Stethoscope* in 2008.

Contributing Authors:

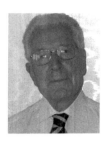

Italo Brambilla, MD started his career in respiratory field in 1970 at Istituto di Fisiologia Umana, Università di Milano, Italy, working with Dr. Emily Milic and director Dr. Emilio Agostoni, in order to specify the diagnostic precocious value of the "closing volume index ". He first heard the name of Dr. Tom Petty in early 1980 when he read the famous paper "NOTT" just published by Ann Intern Med. So, he decided to start long-term oxygen therapy (LTOT) in Italy, having obtained from local health department free use of Liquid Oxygen Portable systems for the first 100 COPD patients with stable chronic hypoxemia. Italian patients on LTOT are 75 000, now. He become convinced of LTOT utility when he read "Prescribing Home Oxygen for COPD" and the next year "Ambulatory Oxygen." So he decided to form an association of patients, with the acronym of AMOR; that is to say *Love.* Now he is going to use the Portable Oxygen Concentrator for some patients on LTOT who need to stay outside home for a time greater than that given by Liquid Oxygen Portable. So they will be able to correct their hypoxemia on a commercial aircraft as well as on long distance trip by train and ship.

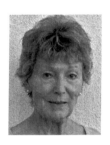

Mary Burns, RN, BS had been working in CCU for 6 years when she very reluctantly agreed to spend just 6 months starting an outpatient pulmonary rehab program. This was in 1975. It took much less time than that to realize that this new field would be the most challenging, rewarding life's work anyone could wish for. Partnering with her patients became an exciting adventure to achieve new and higher levels of activity, and enjoyment in living, for previously depressed homebound patients. She was fortunate to become associated with inspiring, supportive physicians, especially Drs. Tom Petty, Brian Tiep, Rich Casaburi, and Janos Porszasz. Mary feels she was fortunate in her many opportunities to not only welcome visitors to Southern California but to be invited to lecture in their countries. She made good friends while developing a deep appreciation for different cultures and finding all had something important in common. They all wanted to improve the lives of their pulmonary patients. Mary is gradually becoming retired. She is very involved on the Board of her homeowners' association, low water use landscaping, photography and travel. But, she will never stop working with PERF, the Pulmonary Education and Research Foundation, the advancement of pulmonary rehab, or welcoming guests to the Southern California rehab community.

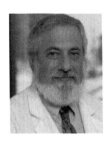 **Richard Casaburi, PhD, MD** is Associate Chief for Research and Professor of Medicine, Division of Respiratory and Critical Care Physiology and Medicine, Harbor-UCLA Medical Center, Torrance, California. He is also Medical Director of the Rehabilitation Clinical Trials Center, a laboratory dedicated to COPD research. Professor Casaburi pursued a research career in biomedical engineering, receiving a PhD from Rensselaer Polytechnic Institute, before qualifying in medicine from the University of Miami School of Medicine. He has authored over 200 publications and 170 abstracts on topics including COPD therapeutics, pulmonary physiology, exercise physiology and pulmonary rehabilitation. One of his career highpoints was co-editing the book *Principles and Practice of Pulmonary Rehabilitation* with Tom Petty

Dr. Casaburi holds the Grancell/Burns Endowed Chair in the Rehabilitative Sciences at the Los Angeles Biomedical Research Institute at Harbor-UCLA Medical Center. He serves as President of the Pulmonary Education and Research Foundation, a non-profit corporation dedicated to advancing the scientific basis and practice of pulmonary rehabilitation. The web site for Pulmonary Education and Research Foundation (PERF) is http://www.perf2ndwind.org/ .

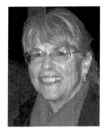

Roxlyn G. Cole, "Lyn," was born and educated on the East Coast and moved to Colorado for the last half of her life. Now retired, she was a YMCA Aquatics Director, involved in writing programs and teaching all ages to 'get and stay fit' through swimming and water exercises. Lyn was diagnosed with COPD in 2003 and this brought about a drive to self educate, learn what caused the emphysema other than minimal smoking. This pulmonary education began my dedication to exercise for better fitness. Testing oxygen related equipment became a passion for Lyn. She has articles published both online and in magazines including *Everything Respiratory, The COPD Digest, AARC Times* and others. Lyn manages a small TTO support group to help those new to transtracheal oxygen systems. She is active with the Colorado COPD Connections group, ALACO Coalition, NHOPA, AARC, CSRC, COPD Foundation and Better Breathers. She also hosts her own "Pulmonary Rehab and After" blog at http://tiny.cc/xglml.

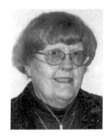

Edna M. Fiore, ASCP was the first Licensed Medical Technologist (ASCP) at the University of Washington School of Medical Technology in 1956. After a 35 year career in Southern California and Oregon as a Medical Technologist/Clinical Laboratory Scientist and raising five children, she became a newspaper reporter, freelance journalist, and historian. Upon retiring in 1996 she joined three of her children in the Conifer area in the Colorado foothills. She is Historian for the Lariat Loop Heritage Alliance and the town of Morrison Colorado, and is working on a book entitled *Saints, Sinners & Stegosaurus*. Edna has been actively involved in COPD Awareness and Advocacy for the past ten years. "The focus of my endeavors in COPD Awareness & Advocacy is to get all of the organizations and institutions 'on the same page' in order to inform the members of Congress and general public about the impact of COPD and the necessity of early detection of COPD, as well as the need for adequate and equitable funding for research and education," stated Edna.

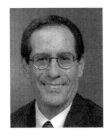

John Goodman, BS, RRT graduated from Stony Brook University in 1972 with a degree in Respiratory Therapy/Cardiopulmonary Technology, and received his credentials as a registered respiratory therapist shortly thereafter. He moved to Denver after graduation, and began working primarily in the intensive care units of several Denver hospitals. He began his teaching career in 1975 as program director at Denver Community College, and has been a respiratory therapy educator essentially uninterrupted since that time. In 1986, he was asked to become director of the Institute for Transtracheal Oxygen Therapy, and was involved in much of the original research that has continued to the present time. John has lectured on transtracheal oxygen therapy in over a dozen European countries, and was named National Honorary Member of the Lambda Beta Society for 2009.

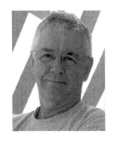

Mark Junge, BA, MA graduated with a B.A. in history and M.A. in Social Studies from Western State College in Gunnison, Colorado. In 1967 he and his wife, Ardath, moved north to Wyoming where they attended the University of Wyoming. In 1972 they settled in Cheyenne where they raised two sons, Andrew and Daniel. At the age of 59 doctors discovered blood clots in Mark's lungs, forcing him to adopt supplementary oxygen. With corporate sponsorship and on behalf of oxygen dependent people he began riding his bicycle across America. Mark is an historian and writer who has authored five books. Currently he is working on another that will detail the 2004, coast-to-coast bicycling experience.

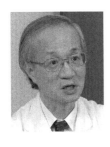

Kozui Kida, MD, PhD started his research career at Postgraduate School of Medicine of Kanazawa University in 1970 where he received his PhD by a thesis of experimental study for lung fibrosis. In 1975, he moved from his alma mater, the Kanazawa University, and started to work at Pulmonary Division, The Tokyo Metropolitan Geriatric Medical Center, Tokyo. From 1978 to 1981, he was working as a lecturer of Pathology Department, the University of Manitoba, Winnipeg, Canada, under the supervision of Dr. William M. Thurlbeck. Whitey Thurlbeck was one of the best friends of Dr. Petty. Kozui first met Dr. Petty in Winnipeg in 1979. After three years research training and his return to Tokyo, Kozui started to work with members of Research Institute of Teijin Co. For 20 years their work on clinical research of oxygen therapy was supported by Dr. Petty and Louise Nett. In 2003, he moved to the present position of professor at Dept. of Pulmonary Disease, the Nippon Medical School, Tokyo, and he published many books for patients with home oxygen therapy in Japan and gave talks to patients directly via radio or TV programs or newspapers.

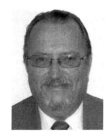

Mark W. Mangus, Sr., BSRC, RRT, RPFT, FAARC has been in respiratory care for nearly 40 years. He started in the field when its presence and scope were experiencing an explosive expansion. He spent 20 years in critical care, 20 years in pulmonary rehabilitation and an overlapping 18 years in home care. Through his work in home respiratory care and pulmonary rehabilitation, he recognized the need to educate and involve resources to improve utilization of this therapy. As an active advisor for EFFORTS (Emphysema Foundation For Our Right To Survive) and columnist for "The Pulmonary Paper" he is able to communicate with thousands of patients with pulmonary disease. Mark runs pulmonary rehabilitation for Christus Santa Rosa at the Medical Center, in San Antonio, a program which he implemented and has nurtured for more than 20 years. He has taught at two local Respiratory Therapist education programs and lectures on several topics, including LTOT and pulmonary rehabilitation. Mark has had the privilege to collaborate with Dr. Petty with The National Lung Health Education Program, EFFORTS and on LTOT issues.

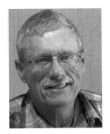

Mike McBride is a Colorado native and grew up in Golden, Colorado. He graduated from Western State College in Gunnison, CO and has lived in the Denver Metro area ever since. Mike was diagnosed with COPD in February 2005 and his response to that news became an obsession to get healthy and stay healthy for as long as possible. His favorite quotes are "they can't bury me if I'm moving" and "I'm sure I'll recognize the limits of my abilities to cope, change, and live well as soon as I encounter them."

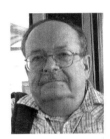

Vlady (Wlodzimierz) Rozenbaum, PhD is the founder and administrator of COPD-ALERT, an online international COPD patient support and advocacy organization, established in 2000 (http://www.COPD-ALERT.com), when he retired on disability from his government job. He has been very active in the COPD community, regularly attending major pulmonary national and international workshops, speaking and publishing about COPD as well as testifying at the FDA hearings and making presentations at the NIH director's meetings. Vlady is a member of the American Thoracic Society (ATS). Vlady is on the Executive Committee of the U.S. COPD Coalition and the Board of Directors of the Pulmonary Education and Research Foundation. He is also on the Editorial Boards of the *COPD Digest* and *Everything Respiratory*. Vlady is a frequent visitor on the Capitol Hill lobbying for COPD patients.

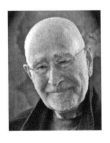

I. Gene Schwarz, MD is Clinical Professor of Psychiatry at the Department of Psychiatry, University of Colorado Health Sciences Center. He is the former Director of the Denver Institute for Psychoanalysis. For the last forty-nine years he has been dividing his time between the practice of psychoanalysis and psychotherapy and the education and training of medical students and graduate mental health professionals both locally and nationally. He has had a special interest in the Law and has conducted seminars for lawyers and judges, as well as being the first psychiatrist to serve on the Colorado Supreme

Court Grievance Committee. At the present time he has become involved in promoting the understanding of the impact of living with Chronic Obstructive Pulmonary Disease and in completing and publishing his second novel. Information on his first novel, *Running on the Edge*, can be found at his web site www.igwrite.com .

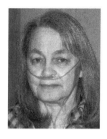

Linda Watson is a 59 year-old housewife, patient, and patient advocate. Her pastimes include gardening and EFFORTS, www.emphysema.net . She lives in upstate New York with her husband, two dogs, and two cats. In 1999 Linda joined EFFORTS and has served on the Executive Board from 2003 to 2008. She has served as President since EFFORTS' founder and president, Gary Bain, passed away in April 2008. Linda says, "We are so honored to have Dr. Petty include us in this book. As a patient, there are not enough words to express what he has meant to us. Thank you, Dr. Petty."

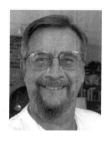

Christopher S. Wigley, BSc, P.Eng was born in England during the war, trained as a mechanical engineer and immigrated to Canada in 1967. I smoked like a chimney and worked in various poor air environments such as an aluminum smelter, sawmill, steel mill and metal forming and machine shops. I got transferred down to Iowa in 1993 and worked until 2002 when I was forced to quit due to health.

Diagnosed with "beginnings of emphysema" in 1993 but ignored this and continued to smoke until about 1998. After I stopped work I started to pay a little more attention to my health and learn about COPD through the Efforts list. I returned to Canada when my wife retired and determined to help those in Canada with COPD. I started a local support group in Duncan on Vancouver Island and then attended the COPD Coalition conference in Calgary in November 2006 (the only patient there!). I joined COPD Canada Patient Network and have acted as Vice-President since it's official start. I sit on the Lung Health Framework Steering Committee attempting to give some direct patient input to their discussions. I hope to continue to serve and promote education and proactive treatment for COPD for as long as I am able.

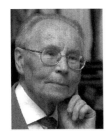 **Jan Zielinski, MD, PhD, FCCP** is a retired chest physician, who, for all his professional life has been attached to the Institute of Tuberculosis and Lung Diseases in Warsaw, Poland. Quite early he became interested in chronic obstructive pulmonary disease, especially in its late complications, respiratory and cardiac failure. Despite the long distance separating Denver and Warsaw, Tom Petty has been for him the mentor and friend. Dr. Zielinski followed Tom's ideas introducing long term domiciliary oxygen therapy and, later, early diagnosis of COPD by spirometry screening in Poland.

"Carpe Diem" does not mean "fish of the day."
— unknown —